Human Well-Being Research and Policy Making

Series Editors

Richard J. Estes, School of Social Policy & Practice, University of Pennsylvania, Philadelphia, PA, USA

M. Joseph Sirgy, Department of Marketing, Virginia Polytechnic Institute & State University, Blacksburg, VA, USA

This series creates a dialogue between well-being scholars and well-being public policy makers. Well-being theory, research and practice are essentially interdisciplinary in nature and embrace contributions from all disciplines within the social sciences. With the exception of leading economists, the policy relevant contributions of social scientists are widely scattered and lack the coherence and integration needed to more effectively inform the actions of policy makers. Contributions in the series focus on one more of the following four aspects of well-being and public policy:

- Discussions of the public policy and well-being focused on particular nations and worldwide regions
- Discussions of the public policy and well-being in specialized sectors of policy making such as health, education, work, social welfare, housing, transportation, use of leisure time
- Discussions of public policy and well-being associated with particular population groups such as women, children and youth, the aged, persons with disabilities and vulnerable populations
- Special topics in well-being and public policy such as technology and well-being, terrorism and well-being, infrastructure and well-being.

More information about this series at http://www.springer.com/series/15692

M. Joseph Sirgy · Richard J. Estes ·
El-Sayed El-Aswad · Don R. Rahtz

Combatting Jihadist Terrorism through Nation-Building

A Quality-of-Life Perspective

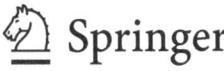 Springer

M. Joseph Sirgy
Department of Marketing
Virginia Polytechnic Institute
& State University
Blacksburg, VA, USA

El-Sayed El-Aswad
Department of Sociology, College
of Humanities and Social Sciences
United Arab Emirates University
Al Ain, United Arab Emirates

Richard J. Estes
School of Social Policy & Practice
University of Pennsylvania
Philadelphia, PA, USA

Don R. Rahtz
Raymond A. Mason School of Business
William and Mary
Williamsburg, VA, USA

ISSN 2522-5367 ISSN 2522-5375 (electronic)
Human Well-Being Research and Policy Making
ISBN 978-3-030-17867-3 ISBN 978-3-030-17868-0 (eBook)
https://doi.org/10.1007/978-3-030-17868-0

This Springer imprint is published by the registered company Springer Nature Switzerland AG
The registered company address is: Gewerbestrasse 11, 6330 Cham, Switzerland

This book is dedicated to our children, grandchildren, great grandchildren, and future generations. The book is also dedicated to all those who have lost their lives to terrorism and to their families, friends, and colleagues who continue to suffer pain from their absence. To all those who gave their lives in the fight against terrorism, and those who, unfortunately, will do so in the future. To those who hold hope that this madness can be deterred and give future generations peace and understanding of their fellow human beings on this earth.

Preface

From M. Joseph Sirgy: Here is a little history to help the reader understand my personal motivation in writing this book. I am a management psychologist (Ph.D. in social/industrial/organizational psychology) and a professor of marketing at Virginia Polytechnic Institute & State University. I have been a professor of marketing for the last 40 years and have written much about quality-of-life issues related to marketing, management, business ethics, corporate social responsibility, public policy, among others.

After the 9/11 terrorist attack in the U.S. (in 2001), several marketing professors (Don Rahtz, Salah Hassan, Jean-Charles Chebat, Barry Babin, Charles Skuba, among others) started exploring the idea that the marketing discipline can contribute to the jihadist counterterrorism academic debate. The marketing discipline seemed so removed from this subject matter, a very important topic to the national discourse. Academics involved in this debate tend to have roots of other social and behavioral science disciplines such as psychology, sociology, anthropology, political science, religious studies, international studies, history, criminology, and military science. Economists, business academics, and marketing scholars, although also social/behavioral scientists, have yet to have made a significant contribution to the growing national discourse on jihadist terrorism and counterterrorism.

An important concept in economics is the market and how market dynamics are influenced by supply and demand factors. Marketing, as an academic discipline, focuses on understanding gaps between supply and demand and how to bridge those gaps. The thought was jihadist terrorism can be viewed as a product (in the same manner we view a consumer good or service) provided by militant Islamists driven by market demand factors. We started to think about these demand factors. What are the demand factors—factors related to religion, culture, governance, economy, technology, globalization, and the media? Using the same lens, we also started to think about supply factors influencing organizational dynamics of jihadist terrorist organizations (e.g., Al-Qaeda and ISIS)—factors related to the marketing of their terrorist campaigns, strategic management, operations, human resource management, financing, accounting, their use of information technology, among others.

Focusing on market demand factors, I realized that many of these factors play a significant role in determining the quality of life of a country. For example, much research in quality-of-life studies have shown that unemployment and religious extremism are negative factors in determining the level of well-being of a country's inhabitants. Overall quality of life of a country is usually determined by assessing the levels of economic, social, educational, health, and environmental well-being of most people residing in that country. A substantial body of research has also shown that those who sympathize and support the jihadist movement in the Middle East and North Africa (MENA) countries and beyond tend to be unemployed and hold extreme religious beliefs. These factors contribute to the market demand of the "service" of jihadist militants. As such, I teamed up with several colleagues (e.g., Richard Estes, Don Rahtz, and Mohsen Joshanloo) to conduct a series of studies to make the case. This effort resulted in several academic publications on jihadist terrorism and counterterrorism.

Professors Richard Estes and Don Rahtz decided that it is time to bring together much of our writing and academic publications on that topic and write a book directed to a broad audience of both academics and practitioners interested in the topic of jihadist terrorism and counterterrorism. Our key goal is to help translate many of the academic concepts and study findings into a language that can be easily consumed by practitioners involved in counterterrorism policy and operations. We then invited Prof. El-Sayed El-Aswad, a cultural sociologist/anthropologist, to join our team. Professor El-Aswad has written extensively on the cultural aspects of the Arab and Muslim world. He is also a native of the MENA region, having spent much time in countries such as Egypt, Bahrain, and the UAE. As such, we thought he would play a key role in guiding us through the Arab/Muslim cultural milieu to ensure that our thinking is indeed grounded in the reality of the region's history, culture, religion, politics, social psychology, and economy.

I also am a native of the MENA region. I was born and raised in Egypt and have spent most of my formative years in Cairo and Beirut. My ethnic heritage is Syrian/Lebanese. Although my parents were not Muslim, I believe I had special insights into Muslim faith and culture because of my formative years. My mother was a Greek Orthodox and my father a Greek Catholic. I completed my primary and secondary education in a parochial Irish (Roman Catholic) school in Cairo. My father's business partner was Jewish, and our families interacted much. As such, I grew up straddling three communities of faith, namely Islam, Christianity, and Judaism.

The impetus behind the book is the fact that much of the literature on this topic (both in the news media and academic journals) have focused on the supply side of the market equation. Much has been written about how to dismantle jihadist terrorist organizations (e.g., how to cut off sources of funding, how to mitigate recruitment of jihadist combatants, how to use technology such as drones in conducting attacks on terrorist suspects, and how to shut down their media outlets) without paying much attention to dealing with market demand factors (e.g., unemployment, religious extremism, lack of political freedom, and lack of cultural diversity). Effective counterterrorist strategies must be based on tackling both sides of the market equation, the supply side plus the demand side. Developing counterterrorism strategies guided by an understanding of the supply factors (conducting terrorist operations, fund-raising to financing operations, recruiting the young and vulnerable, training the recruits, promoting their campaign of terror, etc.) that feed jihadist terrorist organizations is only good for a short term. Yes, we need supply-side counterterrorism strategies to deal with the immediate threat. But dealing with the immediate threat is far from effective. Counterterrorism strategies must also focus on the long term. This is where the demand factors of the market equation come in. This book focuses on understanding market-demand factors of the jihadist terrorism market and proposes a set of counterterrorism strategies designed to reduce future market demand—reduce the risk of future jihadist attacks. Tackling market-demand factors amounts to a strategy that focuses on countries that are most vulnerable to jihadist terrorism in the MENA region and assisting those countries through various institutions (national as well as international) to develop policies and programs to mitigate the risk of future jihadist-inspired terrorism.

We hope that the readers of this book will find the book content useful in the design and implementation of jihadist counterterrorism policies and programs.

From Richard J. Estes: Islam is the world's fastest growing religion and its societies are among the most influential worldwide. But that has been the case for more than 1400 years given that the ancient people of the countries of the MENA region and, in recent centuries, following the death of the prophet in 632 of the Common Era. What became known as "Arabs" in recent centuries were and are people who all share with the rest of the world the beauty of their literature, poetry, song, and dance, the beauty of the Qur'an which builds of the regions other sacred texts, extraordinary artwork, and architecture, and the lingering puzzlements of the Giza plateau which shares the three great pyramids and the much older Sphinx. Arab scientists also gave us a higher quality of paper, the "0" digit that has proven to be so essential to modern mathematics, unparalleled advances in science and technology and, most important for the purposes of this book, a spirit of tolerance for persons of other religious and cultural background. This volume traces an anomaly in the Arab/Islamic communities, that of intolerance, violence, and even terrorism.

All four authors have sought to weave together a coherent history and explanation of the small number of radical Islamists who engage in violence not only in their societies but in those of larger MENA region as well and the world. We believe we have succeeded in achieving our original intention in putting together this book within both a historical and contemporary content.

All four authors also believe that this monograph fills a major gap in the contemporary literature concerning the drivers of violence within and between Islamic communities and other nations. We hope that readers will agree with us on this important accomplishment (along with the rich array of references that also are found throughout the volume).

From El-Sayed El-Aswad: For over 40 years, I have been involved in anthropological studies with a special focus on Middle Eastern and Muslim countries. This focus extends to Arab and Muslim diaspora in the West, particularly the USA. Ethnographic accounts drawn from diverse communities in the Middle East (Bahrain, Egypt and Emirates) and the USA (Dearborn and other places in metropolitan Detroit, Michigan) have provided me with profound insights concerning the patterns of thought and behavior of the people in these communities presented mainly in two monographs: *Muslim Worldviews and Everyday Lives* (AltaMira Press 2012) and *The Quality of Life and Policy Issues among the Middle East and North African Countries* (Springer 2019). The grave problem here is that radicalism and violent actions of militant jihadists have a negative impact on the quality of life and well-being of Middle East and Muslim countries.

Within the quality-of-life framework, this book tackles cultural, religious, economic, political and global media factors underlying drivers of jihadist terrorism to inform long-term counterterrorism policies aimed at not merely reducing or annihilating terrorism regionally and globally but also emasculating the acceptability of violence as a tool for achieving political goals.

For the purposes of theorizing the relation between Islam and radical Islamist jihadism, it is important to draw a distinction between the concept of worldview and that of ideology. The concept of worldview indicates belief systems and related symbolic actions, while ideology, a subcategory of worldview, implies certain economic and political orientations related particularly to power and domination. These two concepts fit the book's main objective seeking to counter the Islamist Jihad' ideological-cultural orientation. In other words, the distinction is crucial for this book as parts of the terrorists' ideology and mission are erroneously assumed by the Islamist jihadists to be related to the worldviews and experience of most Muslims. However, militant Islamist jihadists cling to a narrow and radical view which they try to impose on the rest of the Muslim countries. Muslim scholars refute jihadi radical doctrine or ideology describing it as flawed religious innovation (*bid'ah*). Islamist extremists apply their militant ideology using religious or Islamic concepts, nevertheless they appeal to the minority, not the majority, of Muslims. Policy makers can no longer disregard the threat staged by violent jihadist ideologies and actions, but if they are to be eradicated, they must be identified and understood. Policy strategies and responses to terrorism need to be multi-faceted and efficient. One of the core objectives of this book is to tackle the underlying ideology shared by the jihadist groups, as revealed in their activities and propaganda to provide effective counter-policies for and from governments and civil society both within and without the Muslim world.

From Don R. Rahtz: As a boy, I was an avid reader of any book on history that was in the local library. That obsession with history has stayed with me over the years. As a Southeast Asian major in undergraduate days, I was fascinated by the junction of culture, politics, and religion in shaping the modern world. I found, as many others have, that one could not even begin to understand the world's current with all its trials and tribulations without examining the myriad of underlying historical issues that could create deep seeded affect among players in this endless dance.

Continuing my education in graduate school, I chose Marketing as the business discipline which I soon found had many of the same dynamics as did interdisciplinary degree work in the social sciences. There was a need to understand the underlying drivers for a certain consumer behavior if one was to be able to provide the optimal product/service for a certain group of consumers. Consumer insight came only after a great deal of studying the past experiences of individuals, segments, and even societies and looking for those drivers.

Beginning in the 1980s, I was fortunate enough to have been in the company of a group of interdisciplinary scholars who had been looking at ways in which marketing could make positive impacts on the ultimate quality of life of people not only in a consumer sense, but in all aspects of well-being. For the past 30 plus years, two organizations have been a part of a reshaping of my academic and philosophical approach to research and policy. One of these the Macromarketing Society, I joined after meeting one of its early founding members over coffee and having a heartfelt conversation about "the world and Marketing's role in it." The other organization, The International Society for Quality of Life Studies (ISQOLS) I am proud to have been with it since its creation. This birth came over a conversation on the back porch of a fellow marketer who had also been a mentor to me in my Ph.D. program, Dr. M. Joseph Sirgy. These two organizations approach the world's problems recognizing that the solutions to problems come from an understanding that it is "all connected." One cannot hope to solve the problem without understanding the root causes and trying to connect all the dots. Dr. Roger Layton, a macromarketer, has written extensively about systems and how the macrosystems of markets and societies interact. The mapping and conceptual connections are complex, but if examined closely give insights into how solutions might be uncovered.

Over the years, I have lived and worked in a variety of different cultures around the world and spent a great deal of time trying to gain insights into these cultures. In the latter stages of those travels, it was focused on exploring the quality of life of these cultures and how one might be able to make positive impacts on some dimension of well-being for the people who inhabit those parts of the world. There are paths that can be tested and followed in trying to help mitigate a plethora of underlying drivers of local, societal, regional, and global ill-being. In some ways, I am still that undergraduate trying to figure it all out, who was inspired by many along the way to seeking to provide tools for contributing to a better quality of life for a region of the world that has such a rich and remarkable heritage in every aspect of its being. From Abraham came three great religions that have captured the hearts and minds of so many. I hope that what we have written in the pages of this monograph can aid in helping provide a perspective for all the historical sons and daughters of Abraham to enjoy his legacy in peace. After all, as George Fisk, that early macromarketer had said many a time, "The goal of Macromarketing is to save the world."

Blacksburg, USA   M. Joseph Sirgy
Philadelphia, USA   Richard J. Estes
Al Ain, United Arab Emirates   El-Sayed El-Aswad
Williamsburg, USA   Don R. Rahtz

Acknowledgements

We are grateful to all our colleagues and friends who interacted with us while discussing this important topic. Among them are professors Muzaffer Uysal, Osman Balci, James Littlefield, Reza Barkhi, Manisha Singal, Barry Babin, Jean-Charles Chebat, Salah Hassan, Habib Tiliouine, and Mohsen Joshanloo.

We are also grateful to the editorial team at Springer with special thanks to Esther Otten and Hendrikje Tuerlings. Our special thanks go to the production staff at Springer, particularly Vishnu Muthuswamy. We are equally grateful to our respective families for their moral support and their love. Joe Sirgy's family includes his wife, Pamela Jackson and his four daughters, namely Melissa Racklin (her husband Anton Racklin and her three beautiful children, Isabella, Alec, and Jake), Danielle Gray (and her son Scott), Michelle Sirgy, and Emmaline Smith. A generous thank you also is extended to Joe's two brothers, Abraham and Jimmy and their families, as well as his many cousins and their families scattered in many places around the world.

In addition to thanking one another for the generous amount of time and critiques allocated by the book's author, the remaining three co-authors acknowledge the additional following persons in completing this book: Gail Buchanan Estes, a clinical psychologist engaged in private practice, and wife of Richard J. Estes, and Mariam El-Aswad (a speech and language pathologist), wife of El-Sayed El-Aswad and their sons Kareem and Amir El-Aswad.

About This Book

The first chapter (Chap. 1: In Search of a Roadmap to Peace and Understanding) introduces to the reader a quality-of-life model that addresses the drivers of Jihadist terrorism from which we deduce counterterrorism programs. Specifically, we provide suggestive evidence to show increased incidence of Jihadist terrorism that is mostly motivated by the increased negative sentiment of aggrieved Muslims toward their more affluent Western neighbors. This negative sentiment is influenced by a host of quality-of-life factors: *economic ill-being factors* (e.g., income disparities, poverty, and unemployment; and disparities in technological innovation), *political ill-being factors* (e.g., authoritarian tribal and exclusionary regimes), *religious ill-being factors* (e.g., increased Islamic religiosity, and lack of secularism), *globalization and media ill-being factors* (e.g., the global media), and *cultural ill-being factors* (e.g., perceived decadence of Western culture, and Western prejudice and discrimination).

Chapter 2 (Jews, Christians, and Muslims: Historical Conflicts and Challenges) summarizes the MENA region's rich social, political, cultural, and religious history and brings that history up to the present. We tried to demonstrate that the region's contemporary history of Islamist jihadism and terrorism is rooted in socio-political forces that have been at play for many centuries, indeed, in the case of the region's Jews and Christians, for millennia. These drivers of terrorism, in turn, are based on the high level of grievance that members of the region's three major religions—Judaism, Christianity, and Islam—have endured almost since their establishment. Conflicts with neighboring states, multiple periods of colonial occupation, and the forced displacement of large numbers of the region's people also contribute to the high levels of violence associated with comparatively low levels of quality of life and well-being for a disproportionate percentage of the region's population.

Chapter 3 (Joblessness, Political Unrest, and Jihadism among the Region's Youth: Contemporary Challenges and Future Trends) addresses the major economic driver of Islamist jihadist terrorism, namely unemployment among the youth in the MENA region. This chapter explores the critical relationship that exists between the region's patterns of economic development and its broad-based social gains since the year 2000 to the present. Special attention is given to the relationship that exists between economic frustration, the region's rapid increase in the number of young people, the sense of relative deprivation experienced by these young people and, in some cases, their turning to violence, even terrorism, as an outlet for expressing their frustration and sense of aggrievement toward others they believe to be responsible for their poverty and, more fundamentally, sense of economic anomie.

Chapter 4 (Cultural Drivers of Jihadist Terrorism and Increasing Religiosity) focuses on cultural and religious factors related to the rise of the Islamist jihadist movement. We make the distinction between the Islamic worldview and ideology and place much of jihadist beliefs that motivate terrorist action in the category of ideology. We discuss the cultural drivers of jihadism couched in the context of religious-cultural paradigms. Specifically, we explore cultural and religious factors that drive the behavior or actions of radical Islamist jihadists toward violence, such as grievance and humiliation crisis, revenge and the need to defeat the enemy, establishment of the Islamic State and the re-establishment of the Islamic caliphate, the vanguard of the *ummah*, martyrdom and reward in the afterlife, glorification of Allah, defending sacred places, the temporal paradigm, and chivalric and heroic feats.

Chapter 5 (Political Drivers of Islamist Jihad) focuses on tribal and exclusionary political actions of authoritarian regimes in the MENA. We make the case that those political drivers are associated with Islamist jihadist terrorist actions. We describe the history of authoritarian regimes of Libya, Egypt, Syria, Iraq, Saudi Arabia, and Sudan and jihadist terrorist incidents in these countries. We then concluded with a discussion about Tunisia, a country that experienced authoritarian rule but emerged from this experience with democratic bearings.

In Chap. 6 (Globalization, the Media, and Islamist Jihad), we discuss five major themes directly related to globalization, the media, and their effects on the rise jihadist terrorism in the last 4–5 decades. These themes are (1) globalization and the breakdown of the welfare state; (2) globalization, consumerism, and postmodernism; (3) negative media portrayals of Islam and Muslims in Western and global media, (4) the use of global media by Wahhabis and Jihadi terrorists; and (5) the effects of media owned and operated by political Islamists.

Chapter 7 (Current Response: Counterterrorism Strategies Focusing on the Supply-Side of the Terrorism Market) describes how Western governments as well as governments in the MENA region respond to acts of Islamist jihadist terrorism. The focus seems to be on short-term public safety, or what we call "supply-side" strategies. These are strategies designed to dismantle the marketing organization of militant Islamic groups. Supply-side strategies cannot effectively address the problem of radical Islam without developing compatible demand-side strategies—counterterrorism strategies designed to reduce demand. Thus, demand-side counterterrorism strategies serve to complement supply-side strategies. We tried in this chapter to describe current terrorism policy and action focusing on the supply-side of the terrorism market.

Finally, in Chap. 8 (Proposed Response: Counterterrorism Strategies Focusing on the Demand Side of the Terrorism Market), we recommend counterterrorism strategies focusing on the demand side of the terrorism market. We do so by focusing on drivers of market demand: culture, religion, economy, politics, globalization, and media. We propose specific counterterrorism strategies that are directly deduced from our analysis of the drivers of market demand.

Contents

About the Authors

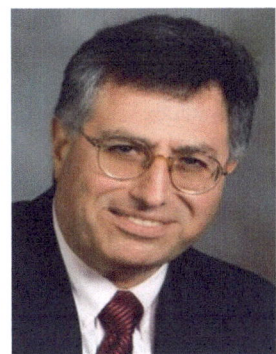

M. Joseph Sirgy is a management psychologist (Ph.D., University of Massachusetts, 1979) and the Virginia Tech Real Estate Professor of Marketing. He has published extensively in the area of marketing, business ethics, and quality of life (QOL). He is the author/editor of many books related to consumer marketing and quality of life. He co-founded the International Society for Quality-of-Life Studies (ISQOLS) in 1995, served as its Executive Director/Treasurer from 1995 to 2011, and as Development Director (2011–17). In 1998, he received the Distinguished Fellow Award from ISQOLS. In 2003, ISQOLS honored him as the Distinguished QOL Researcher for research excellence and a record of lifetime achievement in QOL research. He also served as President of the Academy of Marketing Science from which he received the Distinguished Fellow Award in the early 1990s and the Harold Berkman Service Award in 2007 (lifetime achievement award for serving the marketing professoriate). In the early 2000s, he helped co-found the Macromarketing Society and the Community Indicators Consortium and has served as a board member of these two professional associations. He co-founded the journal, *Applied Research in Quality of Life*, the official journal of the ISQOLS, in 2005; and he has served as editor (1995–present). He also has served as editor of the QOL section in the *Journal of Macromarketing* (1995–2015). He received the Virginia Tech's Pamplin Teaching Excellence Award/Holtzman Outstanding Educator Award and University Certificate of Teaching Excellence in 2008. In 2010, ISQOLS honored him for excellence and lifetime service to the society. In 2010, he won the Best Paper Award in the *Journal of Happiness Studies* for his theory of the balanced life; in 2011 also, he won the Best Paper Award in the *Journal of Travel Research* for his goal theory of leisure travel satisfaction. In 2012, he was awarded the EuroMed Management Research Award for outstanding achievements and groundbreaking contributions to well-being and quality-of-life research. He also edited ISQOLS/Springer book series on *Handbooks in Quality-of-Life Research* and *Community Quality-of-Life Indicators* (Best Practices). He is currently serving as Springer book series co-editor on *Human Well-Being and Policy-Making*.

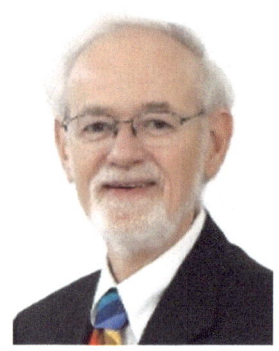

Richard J. Estes is Professor, now emeritus, of Social Work and Social Policy at the University of Pennsylvania in Philadelphia. He holds an A.B. from La Salle University in Philadelphia and graduate degrees in social work from the University of Pennsylvania (Master of Social Work [MSW]) and the University of California at Berkeley [DSW]. He also holds a post-master's certificate in Psychiatric Social Work (PSW) from the Menninger Foundation in Topeka, Kansas. He is a specialist in international and comparative social welfare, social development, and quality of life research. Among other assignments, he has held visiting Professorships in the People's Republic of China, Hawaii, Iran, Kazakhstan, Mongolia, the Russian Federation, Belgium, Italy, Japan, Morocco, Norway, South Korea, Sweden, Switzerland, Mexico, Hong Kong and elsewhere. In the United States, he is the founding President of the Philadelphia Area Chapter of the Society for International Development (SID). He is a former president of the Group for the Advancement of Doctoral Education (GADE) and is a former Chair of the Council on External Relations of the Global Commission of the Council on Social Work Education (CSWE). In 2004, he was elected as President of the International Society for Quality of Life Studies (ISQOLS). He has been the recipient of many awards and research grants, including the prestigious Quality of Life Researcher Award of the International Society for Quality of Life Research (ISQOLS) for his innovative approaches to the dynamics of international social work and comparative social development. In recent years, he has become interested in development patterns occurring in Islamic nations including factors that contribute to Islamic terrorism. He is especially interested in the social, political, economic, historical and cultural roots of jihadist terrorism. He has since written extensively with many Islamic scholars on developing trends occurring in these nations including problems associated with Islamic militancy and terrorism. His publications are quite extensive and include more than 14 books, 100 articles and book chapter, and a long list of radio and television appearances in relation to his research.

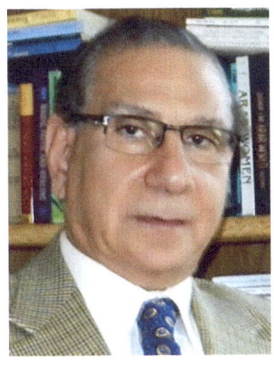 **El-Sayed El-Aswad** received his doctorate in anthropology from the University of Michigan, Ann Arbor. He has taught at Wayne State University (USA), Tanta University (Egypt), Bahrain University and United Arab Emirates University (UAEU). He achieved the CHSS-UAEU Award for excellence in scientific research publication for the 2013–2014 academic year. He served as Chairperson of the Sociology Departments at both the UAEU and Tanta University as well as the Editor-in-Chief of the *Journal of Horizons in Humanities and Social Sciences: An International Refereed Journal* (UAEU). He has published widely in both Arabic and English and is the author of *The Quality of Life and Policy Issues among the Middle East and North African Countries* (Springer 2019), *Muslim Worldviews and Everyday Lives.* (AltaMira Press, 2012), *Religion and Folk Cosmology: Scenarios of the Visible and Invisible in Rural Egypt* (Praeger Press, 2002; translated into Arabic in 2005), *Symbolic Anthropology: A Critical Comparative Study of Current Interpretative Approaches of Culture* (Munsh't al-Ma'raif, Alexandria, 2002) and *The Folk House: An Anthropological Study of Folk Architecture and Traditional Culture of the Emirates Society* (al-Bait al-Sha'bi) (UAE University Press, 1996). He has been awarded fellowships from various institutes including the Fulbright Program, the Ford Foundation, the Egyptian government, and the United Arab Emirates University. He is a member of Editorial Advisory Boards of the Digest of Middle East Studies (DOMES), Muslims in Global Societies Series, Tabsir: Insight on Islam and the Middle East, and CyberOrient (Online Journal of the Middle East). He is a member of the American Anthropological

Association, the Middle Eastern Studies of North America, the American Academy of Religion, and the International Advisory Council of the World Congress for Middle Eastern Studies (WOCMES). He has published 9 books, over 90 papers in peer-reviewed and indexed journals, and over 40 book reviews.

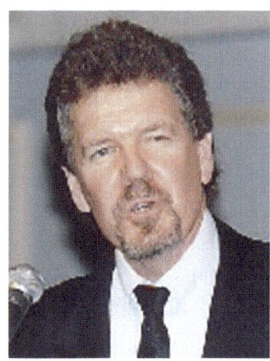

Don R. Rahtz is the J. S. Mack Professor of Business at the College of William & Mary (USA). He has traveled and worked extensively in the developing and transitional world. He has worked on projects in the South Asia, North Africa, and Southeast Asia areas with a focus on Bangladesh, Cambodia, Indonesia, Thailand, and Vietnam. He has conducted a variety of workshops and seminars and acted as a consultant to businesses in both the public and private sectors concerning the above topics, both in the United States and abroad. In addition, he has produced a few publications regarding these topics that have appeared books, academic journals, and the popular press. Don R. Rahtz is a marketing /marketing communications researcher (Ph.D., Virginia Tech 1984) and is the J. S. Mack Professor of Marketing at The College of William and Mary in Virginia. His expertise is in integrated marketing communication programs, international competitive intelligence, cultural intelligence, marketing research, survey methodology, analysis, situational awareness, and market assessment. He has had an interest in Quality of Life (QOL), environmental issues, economic sustainable development, transitional economies, business/community interface evaluation, and health systems. He has served as the Editor of *The Marketing Educator* and on the Editorial Review Boards of *The Journal of Health Care Marketing and The Journal of Business Psychology*. Presently he serves on the Editorial Review Boards of, *Journal of Macromarketing and The Journal of Applied Research in Quality of Life.* He is a regular reviewer for many of the international conferences and journals in the marketing (e.g., Academy of Marketing Science) and quality of life areas (e.g. *Social Indicators Research*). He has published a variety of articles in journals from the social, behavioral science, communication, and marketing areas. His work has appeared in publications such as: *The Journal of Advertising, Journal of Health*

Care Marketing, Journal of Macromarketing, International Journal of Research in Marketing, Psychology and Marketing, Journal of Business Research, The Journal of Applied Research in Quality of Life and *Social Indicators Research.* He has been active in promoting the Quality of Life (QOL) field of study in a variety of disciplines and is a founding member of the International Society for Quality of Life Studies (ISQOLS) where he has served on the Executive Board in several positions and had served as the Vice-President of Programs for over a decade. In 2010, he received the Distinguished Service Award from ISQOLS for his dedicated service to the organization and field. He has served continuously as a Board Member of the Macromarketing Society of nearly two decades and served as the Vice-President of Programs for the society for a decade. He has a long relationship with the International Society of Markets and Development (ISMD) and currently serves on their board.

List of Figures

List of Tables

List of Boxes

Chapter 1
In Search of a Roadmap to Peace and Understanding

Abstract In this introductory chapter, we expose the reader to a quality-of-life model that addresses the drivers of Jihadist terrorism and deduce counterterrorism programs directly from our understanding of these drivers. Specifically, we provide suggestive evidence to show increased incidence of Jihadist terrorism is mostly motivated by increased negative sentiment of aggrieved Muslims toward their more affluent Western neighbors. This negative sentiment is influenced by a host of quality-of-life factors: *economic ill-being factors* (e.g., income disparities, poverty, and unemployment; and disparities in technological innovation), *political ill-being factors* (e.g., authoritarian tribal and exclusionary regimes), *religious ill-being factors* (e.g., increased Islamic religiosity, and lack of secularism), *globalization and media ill-being factors* (e.g., the global media), and *cultural ill-being factors* (e.g., perceived decadence of Western culture, and Western prejudice and discrimination).

Keywords Positive psychology · Quality-of-life intervention programs · Middle East and North Africa · Counterterrorism · Jihadist terrorism · Relative deprivation

1.1 Introduction

In the pragmatist, streetwise climate of advanced postmodern capitalism, with its skepticism of big pictures and grand narratives, its hard-nosed disenchantment with the metaphysical, 'life' is one among a whole series of discredited totalities. We are invited to think small rather than big – ironically, at just the point when some of those out to destroy Western civilization are doing exactly the opposite. In the conflict between Western capitalism and radical Islam, a paucity of belief squares up to an excess of it. The West finds itself faced with a full-blooded metaphysical onslaught at just the historical point that it has, so to speak, philosophically disarmed. As far as belief goes, postmodernism prefers to travel light: it has beliefs, to be sure, but it does not have faith.

Eagleton (2007, p. 10)

© Springer Nature Switzerland AG 2019
M. J. Sirgy et al., *Combatting Jihadist Terrorism through*
Nation-Building, Human Well-Being Research and Policy Making,
https://doi.org/10.1007/978-3-030-17868-0_1

Table 1.1 Terrorist attacks in selected MENA countries compared to worldwide attacks (2015)

MENA country	Total attacks	Total deaths	Deaths per attack	Total injured	Injured per attack	Total hostages
Iraq	3370	6932	2.99	11,856	5.23	3982
Egypt	494	656	1.34	844	1.73	24
Libya	428	462	1.24	657	1.85	764
Syria	382	2.748	7.99	2818	9.78	1453
Worldwide	11,774	28,328	2.53	35,320	3.30	12,189

Source U.S. Department of State, Bureau of Counterterrorism and Countering Violent Extremism. Country Reports on Terrorism 2015. Washington, DC: US Department of State, 2016

Terrorism initiated by a comparatively small group of Islamist fundamentalists remains a global threat. This is particularly true in the countries in the Middle East and North Africa (hereafter MENA), as well as in Western countries, especially those located in the economically-advanced nations of Europe and North America (see Table 1.1). As the table demonstrates, terrorist attacks in the MENA countries has more of its share of terrorist incidents, and most of them are related to Islamist jihadism (see Box 1.1 for a meaning of the term "jihad").

Over the past decades we and our colleagues have sought to better understand this persistent threat to peace and well-being from a myriad of perspectives. Often, the discussions would turn to topics regarding social, political, and economic conditions that exist in Islamic countries worldwide and particularly in the MENA region (e.g., Estes & Sirgy, 2014, 2016; Sirgy, Joshanloo, & Estes, 2018; Tiliouine & Estes, 2016). The conversations and cited research seemed to suggest that these conditions that fostered an almost overwhelming sense of ill-being among many Muslims in the region, especially among those who are not able to participate fully in the economy. We also continued to encounter an apparent linkage of these factors in creating conditions that fuel Islamist militancy both within a militant's country of origin, as well as at the wider regional and global levels. At times there seemed to be a sustained dislike, or even hatred, toward more economically advanced and prospering societies, some of which were former colonizers of the MENA countries.

In building on their own and others past observations and research, Sirgy, Estes, and Rahtz (2017) sought to provide a framework to explore the drivers of Islamist Jihad terrorism (see caveat in Western perception of Islamist jihadism in Box 1.2). They offer a set of recommendations regarding possible counterterrorism measures that are directly deduced from the drivers. Specifically, they provided suggestive evidence to show an increased incidence of Islamist Jihad terrorism is significantly motivated by the increased negative sentiment of aggrieved Muslims toward their more affluent Western neighbors and others who have embraced the Western view of what encompasses success and well-being. This Western view is often framed in the context of materialism and economic well-being being the most important, if not sole, measure of an individual's worth and quality of life. For those who feel ignored or even barred from the opportunities afforded those succeeding in a materialistic and sectarian driven society. A host of quality-of-life factors contribute to a broad negative sentiment. These factors include: *economic ill-being factors* (e.g., income disparities, poverty, and unemployment; and disparities in technological innovation), *political ill-being factors* (e.g., authoritarian tribal and exclusionary regimes), *religious ill-being factors* (e.g., increased Islamic religiosity, and lack of secularism), *globalization and media ill-being factors* (e.g., the global media), and *cultural ill-being factors* (e.g., perceived decadence of Western culture, and Western prejudice and discrimination). This chapter offers a brief primer regarding the pathway by which we will seek to better understand the underlying drivers that seem to contribute to a decade-long state of anger, distrust, and subsequent hatred that has fueled the global Islamist terrorist movement and the call for Jihad against "non-believers" (cf. Khader, Neo, Tan, Cheong, & Chin, 2019). To help the reader understand the path upon which they will follow on this journey the chapter provides an overview of the subsequent chapters and puts forth a theoretical framework that hopefully will provide the reader with a compass by which to better integrate and appreciate the content offered along the journey through the book's chapters.

Box 1.1: What Does Jihad Mean?

The term "jihad," according to the *Qur'an*, means an internal struggle to control one's animal instincts and reform bad habits motivated by these instincts. However, contemporary use of the term has two meanings: the greater jihad and lesser jihad. The "greater jihad" refers to an internal struggle—a struggle that each person has within himself or herself to do the right thing or the moral thing. Doing the right things may reflect a struggle against succumbing to pride, selfishness, and sinfulness. The "lesser jihad" refers to an external struggle that involves the defense of Islam when the community of faith is threatened from those from outside the community of faith (Burke & Norton, 2001, Q&A).

Box 1.2: Not All Muslims Are Terrorists

Most Muslims, even most fundamentalists, are not terrorists. Instead, they have overwhelmingly been the victims of violent conflicts. Hundreds of thousands of Muslims were killed in the war between Iran and Iraq, and the civil wars in Afghanistan and Algeria led to horrific number of casualties. Noncombatant Muslims have suffered untold losses in the war between Chechnya and Russia, in the turmoil in Indonesia, and throughout much of Africa and the Middle East (Kepel & Ghazaleh, 2004).

1.2   The MENA Region and Its History of Violence

Political violence, stemming from religious subjugation and territorial assaults, has been a defining feature of the countries of the MENA well before the introduction of Islam (Cleveland & Bunton, 2016; Donner, 2014; Hirst, 2003). Both the Sumerian and Babylonian civilizations were expansionary in nature and, everywhere, were regarded as fierce warrior societies.

1.2.1   622 CE–750 CE

From its earliest beginnings, as a militant group of soldiers and religious conservatives, Arabs have engaged in conflicts directed against both their polytheistic neighbors as well as those monotheistic believers that did not accept Islam as the true path for entering heaven, i.e., Jews, Christians, and others (Donner, 2014; Kennedy, 2007). This situation eventually pushed Muslims and their non-Muslim neighbors alike into protracted civil wars, with a result of literally hundreds of thousands of persons from both sides of equation perishing in the name of religion.

1.2.2   752 CE–1919 CE

Far from having peaceful relations with their non-Muslim neighbors, these Arab warriors extended their aggression to other regions of the world (Bassiouni, 2016). Among the most dramatic and longest-lasting Muslim conflicts took place in the Mediterranean region of Europe, including the Iberian Peninsula that consisted primarily of Portugal and Spain (Carr, 2009). Arab occupation of the Christian lands of the Mediterranean and the large numbers of people who perished in the related conflicts heightened levels of animosity between Jews, Christians, and Muslims. Eventually, the Iberian population of Christians fell under Islamic control for almost 800 years (from 709 CE to 1614 CE) and served as the model for future invasions by Muslim Arabs into other areas of the Mediterranean as well as Europe more broadly (Kennedy, 2007). Arab-Muslim conquest of still other lands continued after 752 CE until the establishment and eventually collapse of the Ottoman Empire centered in Turkey beginning in 1299 to 1909 (Donner, 2014; Kennedy, 2007). During this period, the Roman Pope and titular head of the Catholic Church, authorized the establishment of the Crusades which, among a variety of other responsibilities, sought to annihilate Arab Muslims and neutralize the impact of Islamic occupations of Christian lands, temples, and other holy sites located in the Near East, but especially Jerusalem (Ashbridge, 2012).

1.2.3 1919 CE–Present

As laid out in the above discussions, the use of violence toward individuals and groups in the MENA region for imposing religious (Islamic, Christian, and Jewish) beliefs, values, and practices from the religion's earliest years to the present time was a frequently-used approach. Although the use of the sword has not been abandoned as a tool for coercing compliance today, much of the contemporary violence is expressed in the form of global terrorism initiated by anonymous terrorists toward anonymous victims.

While historical roots of violence in the region, can provide a broader and, in fact, a deeper understanding of the present, there is a singular event in the region that is often focused on as the catalyst for the emergence of Islamist Jihad terrorism. That event is the establishment of the State of Israel in May 1948. The creation of Israel and, with it, the displacement of thousands of Palestinians from lands that they call home for centuries created an environment in which the seeds of Islamist Jihad and its subsequent terror found fertile ground. The United Nations' Declaration that led to the creation of the State of Israel approved the partition of Palestine into separate Arab and Jewish states and accorded international status to Jerusalem (Cleveland & Bunton, 2016). The claims of Palestinians to their homelands were abrogated by Israel and its supporters[1] with the expectation that neighboring Arab countries would gradually absorb the displaced populations into their own nations (Atiyeh & Hayes, 1992). Most Palestinians, however, continue to live in the region's burgeoning, and deeply impoverished, resettlement camps. As a result, considerable inter-generational conflict persists between Jews and Palestinians. In many situations the conflict has spilled over to the murder of local and national leaders and anonymous citizens of both parties (Jewish Virtual Library, 2018). The return of Jews to what they regard as their historic homeland was further complicated by the emergence of many "Zionists" who emerged at the turn of the 19th century in Europe and who, as a group, have advocated for the return of Jews living in all areas of the world to Israel (Gelvin, 2007). Zionists increased in number and influence following the ending of World War Two in response to the horrific treatment by Nazis and pro-Nazi supporters who systematically persecuted Jews in horrific and unimaginable ways. Zionists have consistently fought for the return of Palestinian lands to Jews, insistent on the exclusion of Palestinians from what are regarded as historically Jewish territories, and consistently have been among the strongest advocates of the State of Israel and its protection. The German extermination of more than six million people during World War Two served as an even greater incentive for Zionists to increase their efforts. At the same time, a rival Arab nationalism also has claimed rights over the former Ottoman territories occupied by the Palestinians, now Israel, and is working to prevent, or at least slow the rate of Jewish migration into the

---

[1]Despite the fact that the United Nations has repeatedly affirmed and re-affirmed that the two-state solution as the only answer to the Palestinian problem (https://news.un.org/en/story/2017/11/637741-day-solidarity-un-reaffirms-two-state-solution-only-answer-question-palestine).

Palestinian territories. These activities have added even more to the covert violent activities taking place in the region (LeVine & Mossberg, 2014).

The contemporary emergence of Islamist Jihad and Islamist Jihadist terrorism focuses on events that have occurred since September 11, 2011—the date when 19 men who were citizens of countries in the MENA region hijacked four fuel-laden commercial jets bound from New York to the West Coast and systemically targeted the destruction the two World Trade Towers (in New York City) and the Pentagon (in Arlington, Virginia). More than 2977 people died in these attacks, including the 19 terrorists—15 of whom were Saudi nationals, 1 Egyptian, 2 United Arab Emirates, and 1 Lebanese (Filote, Potrafkas, & Ursprung, 2016; Freedman, 2010). The attacks were carried out under the leadership of Osama bin Laden, a well-educated Saudi national and in the name of "Jihad." The sections that follow discuss the drivers of this contemporary Islamist Jihadist terrorism in greater detail.

1.3 Understanding the Social Psychology of Islamist Jihad Terrorism[2]

What are the drivers of this contemporary Islamist Jihad terrorism? We have long argued that increased incidence of this kind of terrorism is mostly motivated by increased negative sentiment of aggrieved Arab Muslims toward their more affluent Western neighbors. This negative sentiment is influenced by a host of quality-of-life factors: *economic ill-being factors* (e.g., income disparities, poverty, and unemployment; and disparities in technological innovation), *political ill-being factors* (e.g., authoritarian tribal and exclusionary regimes), *religious ill-being factors* (e.g., increased Islamic religiosity, and lack of secularism), *globalization and media ill-being factors* (e.g., the global media), and *cultural ill-being factors* (e.g., perceived decadence of Western culture, and Western prejudice and discrimination). Understanding the drivers of Islamist Jihad terrorism can help us deduce more effective counterterrorism strategies to reduce this malaise from the MENA region and beyond. See Fig. 1.1.

In the MENA region, developing counterterrorism programs to dismantle existing terrorist organizations seems to be short-term and focuses on the immediate goal of maintaining public order and safety. These counterterrorism programs are short-term because new alternative militant organizations are likely to re-emerge. For example, simply creating a campaign to counter the recruiting call by Al-Qaeda in Iraq reduced recruits for that organization, but the rise of the Islamic State of Iraq and the Levant (ISIL), also referred to as the Islamic State of Iraq and Syria (ISIS), before its recent demise indicated that recruitment remains unaffected. To combat the re-emergence of Islamist Jihad terrorism, public policy and counterterrorism officials within the MENA countries and elsewhere should seek to focus on

---

[2]Much of this section is adapted from our past work, specifically the Sirgy/Estes/Rahtz (2017) article.

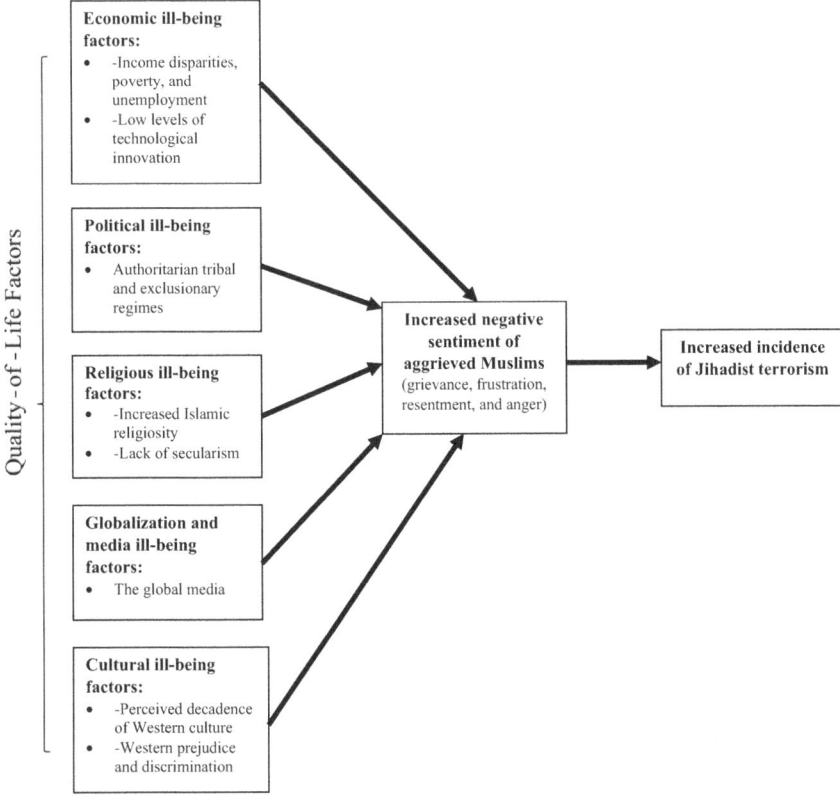

Fig. 1.1 The quality-of-life model of drivers of Islamist Jihad terrorism. *Source* Adapted from Sirgy, Estes, & Rahtz (2017)

the implementation of quality-of-life intervention programs (i.e., programs designed with an eye on the quality-of-life related drivers of Islamist Jihad terrorism). These drivers are related to the economic, political, religious, globalization, media, and cultural conditions that serve as the emotional foundation for the propagation of Islamist terrorism. Central to our understanding of these factors is the notion that marginalized and impoverished Muslims feel aggrieved by predominately economically advanced Western nations. This grievance often activates the process which can ultimately end in an act of terror by a given individual. These perceived grievances and growing frustrations can fuel the terrorism process and motivates the aggrieved persons to acts of terrorism (Chiro & McCauley, 2006; Crenshaw, 2011). To understand the grievance, frustration, and anger experienced by a sympathetic population, one must understand how economic, political, religious, globalization, media, and cultural institutions coalesce to breed this sentiment.

1.3.1   Economic Ill-Being Factors Related to the Rise of Islamist Jihad Militancy

Grievance, frustration, and anger experienced by Muslims, particularly Arab Muslims may be related to economic factors and barriers to opportunity such as income disparities, poverty, unemployment, and disparities in technological innovation. There is a significant amount of evidence that terrorism is linked to poverty (Abadie, 2006; Richardson, 2013). In other words, poverty, relative deprivation, and rapid socioeconomic change can create incentives for people to engage in political violence.

Income Disparities, Poverty, and Unemployment: Income disparities, poverty, and unemployment are all significant factors influencing quality of life of a society. Much evidence in the quality-of-life literature suggest that income disparities play a significant role in quality of life of countries—that is, countries experiencing marked income disparities tend to score lower on quality-of-life measures than countries with less income disparities (e.g., Wilkinson & Pickett, 2009). Similarly, poor countries tend to score lower on quality-of-life indices than rich countries, and unemployment is negatively related to quality-of-life indicators (e.g., Sen, 1981).

Continued and significant unemployment, particularly among youth, leads to a sense of grievance (e.g., Fougère, Kramarz, & Pouget, 2009). Consider the impact of rising unemployment among the youth in Arab countries. The UNDP report (UNDP, 2003) documents the fact that 26% of males between 15 and 24 residing in Arab countries are unemployed. The Arab population registers at 300 million, 37.5% under the age of 15, and three million are in the job market seeking employment every year. The rise of Islamist-inspired militancy is associated with the fact that many Arab countries have large populations of young men who are mostly unemployed.

There is much evidence based on aggregate economic data showing that the MENA region is a global region with most of its population falling below the poverty line (Friedman, 2007). Friedman explains that perhaps one major source of Arab and Muslim humiliation is based on facts like the GDP of Spain—Christian Spain that once was ruled by Arabs and Muslims—is slightly more than the GDP of all the 22 Arab states combined. This fact was addressed by bin Laden as a great insult and source of humiliation for all Arabs and Muslims.

Studies found a positive causal relationship between unemployment and crime rate (e.g., Fougère, Kramarz, & Pouget, 2009). Bayat (2007) states that pervasiveness of unemployment and poverty, along with the rural migration to the cities is likely to provide a footing for major social upheaval. While a variety of studies have fallen short of validating the link between economic distress and terrorism, the general sense is that a combination of political suppression and economic deprivation can foster violence to achieve better economic well-being and enhanced political freedom (e.g., Krieger & Meierrieks, 2011; Kurrild-Klitgaard, Justesen, & Klemmensen, 2006).

With respect to counterterrorism strategies, one may argue that the MENA governments should be encouraged to work toward the development of a wide variety of projects that can employ a significant portion of their young population. It is also important for these projects to span the wide range of skill sets and education levels of the unemployed youth. For example, governments might seek to set up youth conservation corps to put to work more young people in projects focusing on youth development, natural resources conservation, community service, and education to attain skills for success in a modern global environment. In other words, the quality-of-life intervention is to provide economic assistance to aggrieved populations by investing in those regions through projects that benefit the younger population cohorts in a meaningful and sustainable manner. This type of large scale or entrepreneurial focused investment can drive a reduction in poverty. The development and implementation of policies and programs to provide employment opportunities for the youth among the aggrieved public are likely to help reduce the negative attitude toward the offending party, particularly among the youth, which in turn should reduce Islamist Jihad terrorism.

Low Levels of Technological Innovation: There is empirical evidence suggesting a positive link between technological innovation and societal quality of life (e.g., Edwards-Schachter, Matti, & Alcántara, 2012). That is, countries that excel at technological innovation tend to score higher on quality-of-life metrics than countries with a poor record of research and innovation.

Ahmed (1991) offers a "post-modernist" view of the resurgence of Islamic framing of the world. He makes an argument that in the current environment, there is an effort to use "ideal Muslim behavior." In some manner, it is a rejection of a dated "Western Orientalism" view as first put forward by Said (1970) and, subsequently, by a very large number of post-colonial scholars around the world (Tiliouine & Estes, 2016). Said notes that the West continues to create unease and that some Muslims "continue to exhibit a cultural inferiority complex in relation to the West." (p. 224). He seems to suggest that the fall of communism and the embracing of a consumerism-driven society by many from the failed communist regions are inconsistent with Islamic principles. Landis (2015) feels that even the "Arab Spring" of 2011 was driven by western ideals so powerful that they overwhelmed traditional Islamic traditions. It is these collisions of Islam and the West that seem to suggest that Islam may be a moderating force in the acceptance of Western materialism. Given, the rise of global communications and access to technologies and media supported materialism; there may be a growing tension within Islamic communities. Poverty and the size of the youthful populations in most Muslim countries almost certainly is playing a role in a view that is inconsistent between Islam and technology as the West uses it. A savvier and Western-focused segment of the population may view Islam as an "inhibitor of modernization" while others who are trying to apply the brakes to materialism may view technology in a negative manner.

Some data regarding technology and innovation support the notion of disparity between the West and Arab Muslim countries. Based on the second *Arab Human Development Report* (UNDP, 2003), the Arab countries have lagged economically along many fronts. For example, Arab countries produced 171 international patents compared to 16,328 produced by South Korea alone. The average number of scientists and engineers working in research and development in the Arab countries is 371 per million people, compared to the world average of 979. This is surprising given the important, often remarkable and ground breaking, contributions made by Muslims to science, technology, medicine, finance, and literature during its "Golden Age" of the 8th to 14th centuries (Renima, Tiliouine, & Estes, 2016).

Lack of technological innovation and brain drain are problems that are hard to tackle. But that is not to say that these problems are insoluble. An aggrieved population that suffers from lack of technological innovation can learn from India's economic development practices. India has managed to increase its level of product innovation and decrease its brain drain significantly (Friedman, 2007). That country managed to do so by investing in IT education and developing the infrastructure that supports IT firms located in India.

With respect to counterterrorism strategies, this quality-of-life analysis should lead us to conclude that development and implementation of policies and programs to foster technological innovation in aggrieved Muslim countries are likely to help reduce the negative attitude toward the offending party, particularly among political activists. Doing so should decrease the incidence of Jihadist terrorism.

1.3.2 Political Ill-Being Factors Related to the Rise of Islamist Jihad Militancy

Political factors play an important and powerful role in the experience of anger and frustration among the aggrieved. An important example of a political factor that is associated with radicalism and militancy is the prevalence of regimes that are exclusionary and viewed by a variety of groups within the country's population as illegitimate. Political disaffection or suppression can be a key catalyst in both terrorism and civil war (e.g. Kurrild-Klitgaard et al., 2006).

Authoritarian Tribal and Exclusionary Regimes: There is some evidence suggesting that countries with authoritarian regimes score low on quality-of-life indices than countries with democratic regimes (e.g., Dasgupta & Weale, 1992).

A major political situation that seems to have caused much anger and humiliation among Muslims (particularly Arab-Muslims) is the fact that many of the political regimes are authoritarian and suppressive of many freedoms that Westerners take for granted. While two of the most modernized Muslim countries were modernized under authoritarian rule, Turkey and Iran (Farhat-Holzman, 2012), generally authoritarian or single tribal focused regimes restrict widespread plural political participation. Some of those who have legitimate grievances believe that social change can be brought about only through violent means (Crenshaw, 2011). Pargeter (2009) points out that central governments in the MENA region, such as Libya, Morocco, and Tunisia have had a history of marginalizing and even blocking a variety of peoples and regions from any real participation in the process of governing and self-determination. In Iraq, Saddam Hussein brutalized the Shia populations; and in Libya, Muammar Quadaffi did the same to tribes outside of his ruling tribe and supporters. In countries like Morocco and Tunisia, political and economic disenfranchisement, while nowhere near as brutal, was directed by the elites who had consolidated their power in the post-independence environment. When coupled with the creation of many of these countries by Western colonial powers (based on map coordinates or resources instead of historically deep social, political, and ethnic loyalties), the disenfranchisement is not surprising. The effect of lack of political participation in many Arab Muslim countries, government nepotism, and rampant corruption is a recipe for terrorism.

The "Arab Spring" (17 December 2010–December 2012) is a testimony to the fact that anger and humiliation of Arabs and Muslims is partly related to authoritarian, tribal, and exclusionary government regimes. The revolutions in Tunisia, Egypt, and Libya, and the ongoing revolts in Syria, Yemen, and Bahrain reflect this anger. The United States and its Western allies have attempted to effectively advocate for democracy, freedom, and human rights to diffuse the anger that Arabs and Muslims feel towards the West with mixed results. Gul (2012) suggests that the West may need to better understand the role of "secular Islam" in the democracies such as Egypt and Iraq. Sometimes, a Western misinterpretation of secularism can lead to the view that the West is against Islamic-oriented government and would support an authoritarian or despotic choice over moderate secular governments. Lust (2011) points out that individuals, political parties, and governments in the MENA region will also often play on the fear to either keep or usurp power. McCauley and Moskalenko (2011) warn us of "Al-Qaeda's Jujitsu politics" (pp. 156–158). That is, militant groups such as Al-Qaeda and ISIS, in part, justify their violence directed at Western countries because of contemporary Western support for despotic regimes. The more secular regimes (e.g., Bahrain) react (or overreact) to provocations from protestors, the more ammunition militant groups acquire in their *Jihad*.

The preceding discussion seems to suggest that there is a need for governments to temper their tendencies toward a strategy of immediate and harsh retaliation to one that also includes a longer term element that will help address the underlying origins of the protests and acts of violence, One can argue that a counterterrorism strategy for all governments, particularly governments in the MENA region, should include an element that supports the notion of the primacy of human rights and reaffirms the importance of international law. For governments to gain credibility among their own citizens and the international community at large, they should ensure that the political regime in their own countries reflect an open and democratic society. The international community should encourage authoritarian regimes to institute democratic and civil principles, not through force but through education and open dialogue which affirms human rights. In sum, there is no easy answer. It is a very tricky and delicate dance, that will require those involved to work toward the development and implementation of policies and programs to strengthen democratic regimes and transform autocratic regimes into culturally appropriate democratic regimes. We would be remiss in our approach here if we failed to recognize the significant interplay of secular and spiritual aspects in a country's/culture's self-identity, Cultures and countries are defined to a large degree by their political, social, and spiritual foundations. Both secular and religious institutions in countries with an aggrieved populace need to embrace a common goal of well-being for their citizens. In doing so, they are likely to help reduce the negative attitude toward the offending party, particularly among the youth and political activists. Below we turn the conversation toward the spiritual.

1.3.3 Religious Ill-Being Factors Related to the Rise of Islamist Jihad Militancy

Religion has long been recognized by researchers from a variety of the social sciences as something that clearly fulfills the need of many individuals and groups in finding meaning in their identities (Seul, 1999). McBride (2011) recounts the findings of several studies that draw her to assert that terrorist organizations like Al-Qaeda exploit the strength of religion in self-identity and group affiliation by "marrying organizational identification to an over-arching religious paradigm" (p. 565).

Islam is a religion of tolerance, peace, and advancement of good will between Muslims and non-Muslims. The first tenant of Islam is to *submit to the will of Allah* and the will of *Allah*, as revealed in the *Holy Qur'an*, clearly teaches that the level of animosity and violence occurring between Muslims and non-Muslim today is well outside the realm of religious teaching, any religious teachings irrespective of the Islamic domination. Readers should note that there is absolutely no foundation contained in either the *Holy Qur'an*, or the summary of sayings and acts of the Prophet's life, the *Hadith*, that gives legitimacy to the violence taking place by militants under the pretext of Islam, none whatsoever (Keshavjee, 2016).

In effect, Islamic teachings regarding the need for a personal and collective *jihad*, periods of intense reflection and retrospection engaged in by Muslims to improve the religious conduct of their lives, exclude all forms of violence as possible within the religious principles on which Islam is based. Readers also need to remember that the same pattern of inter-faith violence existed during the period of Christian crusades to the Holy Land when Crusaders, operating with the support of Papal mandate, took the lives of hundreds of thousands of Muslims in the name of Christianity or, later, in Catholic Spain and Portugal (the Iberian Peninsula), when the Christians forced both Muslims and Jews to convert to Christianity, leave their countries of birth or, alternatively, die by sword in the name of the Roman Church. The death toll that resulted from this period of the brutal Inquisition is among the least paralleled in other societies anywhere in the world. We offer this brief recounting of the Spanish Inquisition as a reminder here that there is long tradition, one that crosses all religious boundaries, of leaders using a "Jihadist" mindset for political gain.

In today's world, as in the past, two religious factors may be significant in contributing to a rise of anger among an aggrieved populace. These are a rising religiosity and a lack of secularism in a given culture or society. We discuss these two potential drivers of today's Islamist Jihad terrorism in some detail below.

Rising Religiosity: Religiosity (vs. religion) is a complex phenomenon that broadly refers to religious orientation and the degree of personal involvement of an individual with the practices of a religious tradition. According to Cornwall et al. (1986) and Koenig et al. (2005), the concept includes experiential, ritualistic, ideological, intellectual, creedal, communal, doctrinal, moral, as well as the cultural dimensions of personal involvement in religion.

Sociologists of religion have long observed that an individual's religious beliefs, sense of belonging in a religious community, and religious behavior (religiosity) often are not congruent with an individual's actual religious behavior in as much as considerable diversity surrounds a person's degree of involvement in religion (O'Toole, 2001). This contradiction is particularly apparent in Judaism where ethnic identity as a Jew often takes precedence over one's actual degree of involvement in daily Judaic practices (Rosenfeld, 2017). This dichotomy appears to be less extreme among Christians since the period of the Reformation (1517–1648) during which a firm distinction was made between religious and civil society practices (Michalos & Weijers, 2017). The contradiction also is less extreme among Arab Muslims for whom their basic identity and daily activities of all facets of life are inseparably linked to their identity as Muslims.

The subject of religious belief, practices, and religiosity have been the topic of a wide range of quality-of-life studies for decades (Ferris, 2002; Nagpal, Heid, Zarit, & Whitlatch, 2015). Religiosity is negatively associated with country level of development and quality of life. In other words, there is evidence in the quality-of-life literature suggesting that countries with increased religiosity tend to score lower on quality-of-life measures than countries with decreased religiosity (e.g., Barber, 2013).

We believe that a heightened religiosity, driven by core dogma, has a direct and behavior-shaping link with the willingness of individuals to engage in terrorist activities and other acts of aggression that are intended to reduce what are experienced as social pathologies against the targets of their animosity. These targets are often identified as an anathematic outgroup threatening the very core of one's own group social and personal identity. In contrast, increased religiosity, with an increasing closer adherence to Islamic religious teachings and practices (e.g. such as formal worship of Allah multiple times each day, the avoidance of alcohol and "unclean" food), as dictated by Allah (God) through his prophet Mohammed, in turn, can lead to religious extremism that may give rise to radicalism and militancy. As such, Nicholas Wade, the author of *The Faith Instinct*, argues that rising religiosity and warfare are linked (Wade, 2009).

Based on the second *Arab Human Development Report* (UNDP, 2003), the Arab countries have produced only 1% of the books published worldwide. Quite striking is the fact that a large majority of the publications are religious in nature—over triple the world average. This is a possible indicator to a rise of religiosity in the Arab World that works to the exclusion of both secular evidence-based ideas. The Gallup study's examination of the attitudes that constitute the radical extreme (Esposito & Mogahed, 2007) delves into the relationship between the extremists and the Islamic faith they espouse. The study found that while religious rhetoric is closely associated with extremists, and that extremists do give high priority to their spiritual and moral values, the real difference between those who condone terrorist acts and all others is about politics, not piety. Most Muslims, both moderates (90%) and extremists (4%), identify religion as an important part of their daily lives. These facts point to the rise of religiosity in general in the Arab world. Human history is replete with examples of warfare related to rising religiosity.

When couched in the context of counterterrorism, the need for a secular and religious institutional dialogue is again apparent. While a swift and overwhelming, or surgical, military/police strike will remove the immediate or short-term terror threat, the endemic or long-term prospects are not fully addressed without a broad-based secular and religious dialogue. The implication here is that Islamic leaders, referred to as *Imams* or *shaiks*, need to speak more openly about these contradictions between the teachings of Allah, the Islamic Ummah, and the relationship of the Ummah toward their neighbors however different the diverse nature of the people they may encounter are from themselves. They also need to lead their congregations into exploring the true teachings of Islam in relation to such extreme behavior and, in turn, must become active spokespersons leading the way for peace and harmony between Muslims and others (Keshavjee, 2016). A world consisting of more than 1.6 billion Muslims and 1.4 billion Christians cannot move forward without the forceful leaderships of people in both faith communities. In the end, Christians and Muslims worship the same God, pursue the same values and are more like one another than they are different. But the major change that is needed will depend principally on the aggressive teachings of religious leaders of the true tenants of their faith and to make a convincing case to their congregations that their faith has been distorted to achieve unholy purposes.

Another counterterrorism implication of the preceding quality-of-life analysis is to develop programs that introduce, and/or expand existing broader based and secular ideas in Muslim societies that have an aggrieved populace. One way is through science education. The Ottoman Empire. Turkey, Iran, and Iraq all were/are broad based in the study of science and the related arts. Others may involve the study of *comparative* theology and philosophy, creative arts, and human knowledge. In today's world Dubai, Bahrain, and Qatar have all become centers for advanced education in science and the arts through partnerships with a variety of education, medical, and technology leaders and institutions from around the world. The more people become well-versed in science/technology and arts/humanities, the more likely they become less religiously-obsessed. Access to these resources and opportunities across all levels of society are also a critical element in such an approach. One study with national data indicates a negative relationship between level of education and one's religiosity: the most educated are the least religious (Albrecht & Heaton, 1984). That does not mean that they become less spiritual.

Religion and Spirituality need to be distinguished from one another. The better-educated masses (educated in science/technology and humanities) are more likely to feel more spiritual and understanding of the complexity of life. Spirituality is then translated into a personal form of communion with one's own conception of "God." That conception may be divorced from the traditional religious conception.

At the same time, mainstream religions across cultures offer spiritual paths toward the truth. Understanding both classic and modern theology and philosophy provides an alternative religious conception to the radical one. A blind adherence to religious dogma, without an enlightened view of personal spirituality offered in a secularized context can lead to a simple blind view that can, in turn, easily lead to manipulation and exploitation of religious fervor. In sum, one can argue that development and implementation of policies and programs to increase education in science/technology and arts/humanities among aggrieved Muslims, particularly among the youth, are likely to help reduce the negative attitude toward the offending party.

Lack of Secularism: There is some evidence in the quality-of-life literature suggesting that secularism is associated with quality-of-life indicators (e.g., Li & Bond, 2010). In other words, countries that are more secular (less religious) tend to score higher on quality-of-life indices than countries that are less secular.

Lack of secularism in certain inward-looking Muslim countries may play a significant role in the rise of radicalism and militancy in those countries. For example, Wade (2009) also points to the notion that Qur'anic discussion of warfare is directly associated with the joys of paradise, which further justifies and encourages violence. While the Western view may be that there is no separation of religion and state in Islamic countries, the interpretation of how embedded Islam is and how meshed it is with the state is one that is misunderstood (Gul, 2012). "The idea that any group of persons, any activities, any part of human life is in any sense outside the scope of religious law and jurisdiction is alien to Muslim thought," writes Bernard Lewis (2002, p. 100), a leading scholar of Islam. While this quote would lead many in the West to believe that any nation that has an Islamic government is not secular, there are many scholars who have examined the topic and report that such a "blanket" statement or view fails to address the wide variance and application of Islamic-oriented democracy. Hefner (2014a, 2014b) provides support for a historical Islam that was steeped in diversity and plurality.

It follows that policies that encourage some sort of demarcation between religion and the State should be encouraged. That is not to say that a strict application of a Western view of the separation of "Mosque and State" should be strongly advocated. Some Islamic states in the MENA region use the *Shari'a* as their only or primary source of law. Reformers in the Muslim world have met much resistance from the religious clerics who continue to exercise their power of persuasion on the public. Separation of religion from the State is perceived as a Western liberal concept by many Muslim clerics (Huntington, 1993). There are many anecdotes of failures of reform to separate religion from state, the most recent examples are in Iran and Turkey. Secular Arab countries such as Egypt, Syria, Algeria, and Yemen are struggling to maintain their foothold of power. Radical Islamist fundamentalist movements in these countries push hard for a restoration of Islamic rule and pose a serious threat to the stability of secular governments (Fox & Sandler, 2005).

Although secularization efforts are used by radical Islamist fundamentalists as rallying points in opposition to secularization (e.g., ISIS) the counterterrorism quality-of-life implication is to develop programs that promote secularism with a clear eye on benefits gained from such a path. That is, development and implementation of policies and programs to promote a culturally sensitive secularism in Muslim countries with an aggrieved public are likely to help reduce Islamist Jihadist terrorism.

1.3.4 Globalization and Media Ill-Being Factors Related to the Rise of Islamist Jihad Terrorism

Globalization can bring about marginalization when countries fall behind in delivering a standard of living below the norm, in which the norm is clearly publicized through the global media (e.g., Sirgy, 1998; Sirgy et al., 1998). In other words, the marginalized people become acutely aware of their backwardness by witnessing the standard of living (and potentially the perceived decadence and political indifference) of the developed Western and Western-oriented world. This is exactly what happened to many of the less-developed Arab and Muslim countries (Friedman, 2007). Arabs and Muslims have felt an increasing sense of social alienation and a sense of humiliation at their comparative backwardness in the broader globalized society and economy. Globalization and the widespread dissemination of media have allowed the entire Islamic world to observe and be involved in the debate. As media have delivered a constant stream of content, Arabs observed their descent from a great Islamic civilization to a world of underdevelopment. History shows that they had a great sense of pride in their Arab and Muslim identity; now they seem to have lost that sense of pride. The media have played a significant role in the promulgation of these feelings of dissonance and dislocation.

The Global Media: Friedman (2007) has argued that globalization serves to create greater flow among people and cultures. In other words, globalization breaks down barriers among people of different nationalities and culture. Globalization connects people to people. Thus, people become increasingly aware of other people and their culture. The effect of globalization on cultural awareness is positive to some people but negative to others. The real war is not so much about what goes on it the West, but how Muslim governments are now corrupted from their ideals. Global media, however, often plays a role in highlighting the negatives of Islamic countries on broadcasts and a variety media platform from the internet and mobile social media. Ciftci (2012) notes that Islamophobia has reached unprecedented levels in the West. Much of that message of all Arabs are backwards, inferior, fanatical, and violent finds its way onto platforms viewed by the Arab World. Donald Trump's advocacy for "banning all Muslims" from coming to the United States was posted in Islamic country media almost immediately. It also found its way into recruitment videos for ISIS. In such a global media environment, many Muslims around the world, especially Arab-Muslims feel frustrated and humiliated by the awareness of how the West has treated them both currently and throughout history; and according to Friedman, this perception may have contributed to the rise of the suicide bombers of Al-Qaeda and other Islamist terror organizations.

Furthermore, according to Friedman (2007), globalization has made the backwardness of the Arab-Muslin world (compared to the Western world), hard to ignore. Arab-Muslim intellectuals have consistently demanded solutions from their political leaders by pointing to this backwardness. This perceived backwardness has been a great source of humiliation and loss of pride among Muslims and Arabs. The notion of restoring the Caliphate is an emotional appeal to rebuild a rival civilization to that of the Western civilization and create a major source of pride and honor to all Arabs and Muslims worldwide. A contributing factor to this problem is the lack of awareness and appreciation among broad Western audiences of the major contributions of Islamic civilization to science and arts over history (Stearns, 2014). At the same time, there is a mythical view held by Islamists of an Islamic Golden Age (Al-Andalus in the Middle-Ages) that flourished until it was brutally destroyed by the colonization of Islamic lands by the Western powers. While there was a flourishing culture in parts of MENA region, the "Golden Age" had long been in decline. There were still tribal conflicts, and a variety of social ills before Western colonization. In a post-colonial environment, the failure to achieve a return to the mythical "Golden Age" contributed to a level of enhanced mythical proportions. A key point to note here as well, is that in this environment of unmet expectations, Islamists use of the West as the reason for failure. This further contributes to the epic narrative. Githens-Mazer (2008) points out this perceived "injustice" combined with a view that it was done with "contempt" to "humiliate" a flourishing culture is a key element in radicalization.

With respect to counterterrorism, the same forces of globalization that have served to propagate the image of "backwardness" of the aggrieved population can be used to highlight and publicize progress and achievements. The plethora of media platforms and outlets can mitigate these negative feeling through an emphasis on what the aggrieved population has contributed to modern society (Maziak, 2005). Consider the following example. In 2008, a science exhibition was held at the University of Sharjah (U.A.E) called "Sultans of Science Rediscovered." The exhibition covered Arab and Muslim scientific achievements in architecture, arts, astronomy, engineering, exploration, flight, mathematics, medicine, optics, fine and utilitarian technology, and water control (http://www.adach.ae/en/default.aspx). The conference recognized Muslims' scientific achievements. The same venue was used to develop an agenda for next steps for future advancements in science and technology in MENA countries (AMEinfo.com, 2008). This is very important in that not only can science and technology help create wealth, but they can help reduce societal tensions and build international bridges for badly needed dialogue and mutual understanding (Maziak, 2005). Dubai, for example, is often cited for its technological and architectural leadership on the global stage, in sum, development and implementation of policies and programs to publicize political, cultural, scientific, and technological achievements, particularly in global media, are likely to help reduce Jihadist terrorism.

1.3.5 Cultural Ill-Being Factors Related to the Rise
of Islamist Jihad Militancy

Culture plays an important role in the festering of anger and negative feelings of an aggrieved public toward an offending party. For example, Friedman (2007) has argued that there is a host of cultural factors that have contributed to the festering of anger and humiliation among Muslims, particularly Arab Muslims. These are related to the perception that Western culture is decadent, and the manifest prejudice and discrimination leveled against Muslim immigrants in the West.

Perceived Decadence of Western Culture: There is some evidence in the quality-of-life literature suggesting that Islamic societies that reject modernity and adhere to Islamic law tend to report lower levels of quality of life (e.g., Estes & Sirgy, 2014). Modernity can be construed as reflective of Western culture. Hence, Muslim countries that reject modernity are likely to experience lower levels of well-being, compared to countries embracing modernity.

Typically, terrorist groups view the offending party in the most negative terms. The offending party is the enemy, decadent, and evil. A major impetus to restore the Caliphate is the frustration that Arab Muslims feel in observing the lifestyle of Westerners, and especially how this lifestyle is influencing their own youth. When Muslim fundamentalists look at the West they see evil—a culture of decadence and promiscuity. Restoring the Caliphate is a means to replace a decadent culture with a moral one—not only for all Arabs and Muslims but for the entire of humanity (Friedman, 2007). In a Gallup poll conducted in nine Muslim countries in December 2001 and January 2002, most respondents indicated that they considered the United States to be evil in terms of being ruthless, arrogant, aggressive, and a *corrupting influence* (Blaydes & Linzer, 2012). Shafiq (2009) examined data from the 2005 Pew Project and found that both education and income have a significant influence in people's support for democracy in Muslim countries.

The counterterrorism implication in this case is to identify the exact nature of the negative image of the offending party and create a well-researched, broad based, multi-media promotion campaigns to pull back the curtain of misunderstanding to help change this image in the minds of the aggrieved party. This campaign must be one that truthfully addresses the concerns of all relevant publics and segments. Much of the work on "in-group versus out-group behavior" from sociology and social psychology (e.g., Costarelli, & Gerłowska, 2015) can be molded to help address this problem. Promotion campaigns should focus on "humanizing" the offending party by highlighting societal problems and showing how responsible and moral leaders are dealing with these problems in human terms. That is, development and implementation of policies and programs to promote the offending party as "human" afflicted with human problems and trying to deal with these problems through responsible and moral leadership are likely to help reduce Jihadist terrorism.

Western Prejudice and Discrimination: There is much evidence suggesting that immigrants who experience prejudice and discrimination are likely to experience lower levels of life satisfaction than those who experience less prejudice and discrimination (Safi, 2009). In today's world of global social media connectedness, sharing that prejudice and discrimination experience with a broad audience in almost or actual real-time is easy. Many of the immigrants communicate their negative experiences in their host countries to their friends and relatives in their home countries. Again, consider the case of the Arabs and Muslims who perceive prejudice and discrimination. Many Arabs and Muslims, having immigrated to Western countries (or having grown up in the West), feel very alienated because of their efforts to maintain their own Islamic culture. A study by Fischer et al. (2007) found that Muslims in Germany were not more aggressive than Christians and secular westerners (as perceived by the westerners) but were concerned that Western societies were threatening their religious identity through various actions (e.g. no headscarves in schools, etc.). This perceived threat to religious identity was found to be a driver in the creation of a different "attitude toward terrorism." Unfortunately, this may well lead some to view this as an affirmation of the stereotype held by the Westerners.

There have been many incidences of Western expression of prejudice and discrimination against Muslims in places like the U.S., the U.K., France, and Germany. An example of this prejudice is the 2007 referendum in Switzerland that resulted in a vote against building minarets. The result is a feeling of rejection—a feeling that "you are not one of us." This sense of alienation quickly turns to humiliation, anger, and rage, which in turn make Arab and Muslim youth highly receptive to the persuasive message of terrorist groups and their recruiting disciples (Friedman, 2007). McCauley and Moskalenko (2011) warn us how militant groups such as Al-Qaeda use "minor provocations" (e.g., the failed Nigerian terrorist, Umar Farouk Abdulmutallab, the "Underwear Bomber") to their advantage. Typically, minor provocations induce public policy officials to overreact by creating policies and programs that exacerbate prejudice and discrimination directed at the Arab-Muslim community (e.g., new visa restrictions, profiling at airports, overzealous law enforcement agents arresting, and interrogating Arab-Muslims based on "atypical" behaviors or very minor offenses). Such manifestations of prejudice and discrimination are further used by militant groups to promote their *Jihad*.

The counterterrorism implications in this case must be the enforcement of all laws related to prejudice and discrimination as well as cultural awareness. Inclusiveness and sensitivity training in all sectors of society. One can observe many years of progress made in U.S. race relations and civil rights of Arabs and Muslims immigrants in the West. Also, for any progress to be realized, "offending" countries must promote policies that encourage educational and cultural exchange programs with the aggrieved parties. In sum, development and implementation of policies and programs to reduce prejudice and discrimination toward the aggrieved party is likely to help reduce Islamist Jihadist terrorism.

1.4   Conclusion

If strategically directed quality-of-life intervention programs can work to diminish this feeling and reduce the percentage of the politically radicalized, this could lead to a significant reduction in Islamist Jihadist terrorism. Combating terrorism using military force to dismantle terrorist organizations can be viewed as short-term and short-sided solution. It is best to focus on the big picture that explains the drivers for terrorism and implement quality-of-life intervention programs to reduce Islamist Jihadist terrorism.

In the pages that follow in this book we expand our search for a roadmap to give the reader a better understanding of the causes of Islamist Jihadist Terrorism, It is a roadmap built upon a quality-of-life framework that seeks to recognize the problem within the context of an interconnected and broad-based system that not only exists within a local network and within a global network, but across these networks as well. To borrow from a well-known advertising pitch for Las Vegas, "What happens locally, does not stay locally. It goes global as well and ultimately returns to the local with global implications. Chapter two begins our journey at the point of origin and the Father of nations Abraham.

References

Abadie, A. (2006). Poverty, political freedom, and the roots of terrorism. *American Economic Review, 96,* 50–56.

Ahmed, A. S. (1991). Postmodernist perceptions of Islam: Observing the observer. *Asian Survey, 31,* 213–231.

Albrecht, S. L., & Heaton, T. B. (1984). Secularization, higher education, and religiosity. *Review of Religious Research, 26,* 43–58.

AMEinfo.com. (2008, March 31). Arab and Muslim science legacy on tour. *AMEinfo.com.* http://www.ameinfo.com/151814.html.

Ashbridge, T. (2012). *The Crusades: The war for the holy land.* New York: Simon & Schuster.

Atiyeh, G. N., & Hayes, J. R. (1992). *The genius of Arab civilization.* New York: New York University Press.

Barber, N. (2013). Country religiosity declines as material security increases. *Cross-Cultural Research, 47,* 42–50.

Bassiouni, C. M. (2016). Islam and contemporary radicalized violence: A historic turning point. In R. J. Estes & H. Tiliouine (Eds.), *Social progress in Islamic societies: Social, political, economic, and ideological challenges* (pp. 547–573). Dordrecht NL: Springer.

Bayat, A. (2007). Radical religion and the habitus of the dispossessed: Does Islamic militancy have an urban ecology? *International Journal of Urban and Regional Research, 31,* 579–590.

Blaydes, L., & Linzer, D. A. (2012). Elite competition, religiosity, and anti-Americanism in the Islamic World. *The American Political Science Review, 106,* 225–243.

Burke, J., & Norton, J. (2001, October 4). Islamic fundamentalism: A world-renowned scholar explains key points of Islam. *Christian Science Monitor.* (Q&A).

Carr, M. (2009). *Blood and faith: The purging of Muslim Spain.* New York: The New Press.

Chiro, C., & McCauley, C. (2006). *Why not kill them all? The logic and prevention of mass political murder.* Princeton, NJ: Princeton University Press.

Ciftci, S. (2012). Islamophobia and threat perceptions: Explaining anti-Muslim sentiment in the West. *Journal of Muslim Minority Affairs, 32,* 293–309.

Cleveland, W. L., & Bunton, M. (2016). *A history of the modern Middle East* (6th ed.). Boulder: Westview Press.

Cornwall, M., Albrecht, S. L., Cunningham, P. H., & Pitcher, B. L. (1986). The dimensions of religiosity: A conceptual model with an empirical test. *Review of Religious Research, 27,* 226–244.

Costarelli, S., & Gerłowska, J. (2015). Ambivalence, prejudice and negative behavioural tendencies towards out-groups: The moderating role of attitude basis. *Cognition and Emotion, 29,* 852–866.

Crenshaw, M. (2011). *Explaining terrorism: Causes, processes and consequences.* New York: Routledge.

Dasgupta, P., & Weale, M. (1992). On measuring the quality of life. *World Development, 20,* 119–131.

Donner, F. M. (2014). *The early Islamic conquests.* Princeton NJ: Princeton University Press.

Eagleton, T. (2007). *The meaning of life.* New York: Barnes and Noble.

Edwards-Schachter, M. E., Matti, C. E., & Alcántara, E. (2012). Fostering quality of life through social innovation: A living lab methodology study case. *Review of Policy Research, 29,* 672–692.

Esposito, J., & Mogahed, D. (2007). *Who speaks for Islam? What a billion Muslims really think?.* Washington, DC: Gallup Press.

Estes, R. J., & Sirgy, M. J. (2014). Radical Islamic militancy and acts of terrorism: a quality-of-life analysis. *Social Indicators Research, 117,* 615–652.

Estes, R. J., & Sirgy, M. J. (2016). Is quality of life related to radical Islamic militancy and acts of terrorism? In R. J. Estes & H. Tiliouine (Eds.), *Social progress in Islamic Societies: Social, political, economic, and ideological challenges* (pp. 575–605). Dordrecht NL: Springer.

Farhat-Holzman, L. (2012). Modernization or westernization: the Muslim world vs. the rest. *Comparative Civilizations Review, 67,* 50–62.

Ferris, A. (2002). Religion and the quality of life. *Journal of Happiness Studies, 3,* 199–215.

Filote, A., Potrafke, N., & Ursprung, H. (2016). Suicide attacks and religious cleavages. *Public Choice, 166,* 3–28.

Fischer, P., Greitemeyer, T., & Kastenniüller, A. (2007). What do we think about Muslims? The validity of Westerners' implicit theories about the associations between Muslims' religiosity, religious identity, aggression potential, and attitudes toward terrorism. *Group Processes & Intergroup Relations, 10,* 373–382.

Fougère, D., Kramarz, F., & Pouget, J. (2009). Youth unemployment and crime in France. *Journal of the European Economic Association, 7,* 909–938.

Fox, J., & Sandler, S. (2005). Separation of religion and State in the twenty-first century: Comparing the Middle East and Western Democracies. *Comparative Politics, 37,* 317–335.

Freedman, B. (2010). *Perspectives on terrorism: Terrorism research centres* (vol. 4, no. 5). University of Leiden (Netherlands), Terrorism Research Initiative (TRI). Retrieved May 15, 2017 from http://www.terrorismanalysts.com/pt/index.php/pot/article/view/123/html.

Friedman, T. L. (2007). *The world is flat.* New York: Picador.

Gelvin, J. (2007). *The Israel–Palestine conflict: One hundred years of war* (2nd ed.). Cambridge University Press.

Kepel, G., & Ghazaleh, P. (2004). *The war for Muslim minds: Islam and the West* (p. 256). Cambridge, MA: Belknap Press of Harvard University Press.

Githens-Mazer, J. (2008). Islamic radicalization among North Africans in Britain. *British Journal of Politics & International Relations, 10,* 550–570.

Gul, A. (2012). Egyptian Muslims should embrace secularism. *NPQ: New Perspectives Quarterly, 29,* 48–51.

Hefner, R. (2014a). Islam and plurality, old and new. *Society, 51,* 636.

Hefner, R. (2014b). Modern Muslims and the challenge of plurality. *Society, 51,* 131.

Huntington, S. P. (1993). The clash of civilizations? *Foreign Affairs, 72,* 22–49.

Hirst, D. (2003). *The gun and the olive branch: The roots of violence in the Middle East* (3rd ed.). New York: Nation Books.

Jewish Virtual Library. (2018). *Vital statistics: Total casualties, Arab-Israeli conflict—1849–present*. Retrieved March 14, 2018 from http://www.jewishvirtuallibrary.org/total-casualties-arab-israeli-conflict.

Kennedy, H. (2007). *The great Arab conquests: How the spread of Islam changed the world we live in*. Boston: De Capo Press.

Keshavjee, M. (2016). Alternate dispute resolution (ADR) and its potential for helping Muslims resolve the high ethical values underpinning Sharia. In H. Tiliouine & R. J. Estes (Eds.), *Social progress in the Islamic world: Social political, economic, and ideological challenges* (pp. 607–621). Dordrecht NL: Springer.

Khader, M., Neo, L. S., Tan, J., Cheong, D. D., & Chin, J. (2019). *Learning from violent extremist attacks: Behavioural sciences insights for practitioners and policymakers*. New Jersey: World Scientific/WorldSciNet.

Koenig, L. B., McGue, M., Krueger, R. F., & Bouchard, T. J. (2005). Genetic and environmental influences on religiousness: Findings for retrospective and current religiousness ratings. *Journal of Personality, 73*, 471–488.

Krieger, T., & Meierrieks, D. (2011). What causes terrorism? *Public Choice, 147*, 3–27.

Kurrild-Klitgaard, P., Justesen, M. K., & Klemmensen, R. (2006). The political economy of freedom, democracy and transnational terrorism. *Public Choice, 128*, 289–315.

Landis, B. (2015). The Islamic world faces its future. *American Diplomacy*, 19–28.

LeVine, M., & Mossberg, M. (2014). *One land, two states: Israel and Palestine as parallel states*. Berkeley: University of California Press.

Lewis, B. (2002). *What went wrong? The clash between Islam and modernity in the Middle East*. New York: Harper-Collins.

Li, L. M. W., & Bond, M. H. (2010). Does individual secularism promote life satisfaction? The moderating role of societal development. *Social Indicators Research, 99*, 443–453.

Lust, E. (2011). Missing the third wave: Islam, institutions, and democracy in the Middle East. *Studies in Comparative International Development, 46*, 163–190.

Maziak, W. (2005). Science in the Arab World: Vision of glories beyond. *Science, 308*, 1416–1418.

McBride, M. K. (2011). The logic of terrorism: Existential anxiety, the search for meaning, and terrorist ideologies. *Terrorism and Political Violence, 23*, 560–581.

McCauley, C., & Moskalenko, S. (2011). *Friction: Radicalization happens to them and us*. New York: Oxford University Press.

Michalos, A. C., & Weijers, D. (2017). Western historical traditions of well-being. In R. J. Estes & M. J. Sirgy (Eds.), *The pursuit of human well-being: The untold global history* (pp. 31–58). Dordrecht NL: Springer.

Nagpal, N., Heid, A. R., Zarit, S. H., & Whitlatch, C. J. (2015). Religiosity and quality of life: A dyadic perspective of individuals with dementia and their caregivers. *Aging Mental Health, 19*, 500–506.

O'Toole, R. (2001). Sociology of religion. In: *International encyclopedia of the social & behavioral sciences* (pp. 13106–13112). Amsterdam: Elsevier.

Pargeter, A. (2009). Localism and radicalization in North Africa: local factors and the development of political Islam in Morocco, Tunisia and Libya. *International Affairs, 85*, 1031–1044.

Renima, A., Tiliouine, H., & Estes, R. J. (2016). The Islamic golden age: A story of the triumph of the Islamic civilization. In H. Tiliouine & R. J. Estes (Eds.), *The state of social progress of Islamic societies: Social, political, economic, and ideological challenges* (pp. 24–52). Dordrecht NL: Springer.

Richardson, L. (2013). *The roots of terrorism*. London: Routledge.

Rosenfeld, M. (2017). Secular Jewishness; what's Jewish about it? Retrieved October 20, 2017 from http://www.csjo.org/resources/essays/secular-jewishness-whats-jewish-about-it/.

Safi, M. (2009). Immigrants' life satisfaction in Europe: Between assimilation and discrimination. *European Sociological Review, 26*, 159–176.

Said, E. (1970). *Orientalism*. New York: Vintage.

Sen, A. (1981). Public action and the quality of life in developing countries. *Oxford Bulletin of Economics and Statistics, 43,* 287–319.

Seul, J. R. (1999). 'Ours is the way of god': Religion, identity, and intergroup conflict. *Journal of Peace Research, 36,* 553–569.

Shafiq, M. N. (2009). *Do education and income affect support for democracy in Muslim countries? Evidence from the "Pew Global Attitudes Project."* Online Submission.

Sirgy, M. J. (1998). Materialism and quality of life. *Social Indicators Research, 43,* 227–260.

Sirgy, M. J., Estes, R. J., & Rahtz, D. R. (2017). Combatting jihadist terrorism: A quality-of-life perspective. *Applied Research in Quality of Life.* https://doi.org/10.1007/s11482-017-9574-z. (in press)

Sirgy, M. J., Joshanloo, M., & Estes, R. J. (2018). The global challenge of Jihadist terrorism: A quality-of-life model. *Social Indicators Research,* https://doi.org/10.1007/s11205-017-1831-x. (in press).

Sirgy, M. J., Lee, D. J., Kosenko, R., Lee Meadow, H., Rahtz, D., Cicic, M., et al. (1998). Does television viewership play a role in the perception of quality of life? *Journal of Advertising, 27,* 125–142.

Stearns, J. (2014). All beneficial knowledge is revealed: The rational sciences in the Maghrib in the age ofal-Yūsī (d. 1102/1691). *Islamic Law & Society, 21,* 49–80.

Tiliouine, H., & Estes, R. J. (2016). *Social progress in the Islamic world: Social political, economic, and ideological challenges.* Dordrecht: Springer.

United Nations Development Programme (UNDP). (2003). *The Arab human development report.* New York: Oxford University.

Wade, N. (2009). *The faith instinct: How religion evolved and why it endures.* New York: The Penguin Press.

Wilkinson, R. G., & Pickett, K. (2009). *The spirit level: Why more equal societies almost always do better* (Vol. 6). London: Allen Lane.

Chapter 2
Jews, Christians, and Muslims: Historical Conflicts and Challenges

Abstract This chapter summarizes the MENA region's rich social, political, cultural, and religious history and brings that history up to the present. The purpose of this summary is to demonstrate that the region's contemporary history of Islamist jihadism and terrorism is rooted in socio-political forces that have been at play for many centuries, and indeed, in the case of the region's Jews and Christians, for millennia. These drivers of terrorism, in turn, are based on the high level of grievance that members of the region's three major religions—Judaism, Christianity, and Islam—have endured almost since their establishment. Conflicts with neighboring states, multiple periods of colonial occupation, and the forced displacement of large numbers of the region's people also contribute to the high levels of violence associated with comparatively low levels of quality of life and well-being for a disproportionate percentage of the region's population.

Keywords History of Islam · Islamist jihadism · Judaism · Christianity · Islam · Religious conflict

2.1 Introduction

> "Abram fell on his face, and God talked with him, saying, "As for Me, behold, My covenant is with you, and you will be the father of a multitude of nations." No longer shall your name be called Abram; but your name shall be Abraham; for I have made you the father of a multitude of nations." Genesis 17:3-6

The MENA region historically is one of the world's most influential centers of human civilization. Unfortunately, and despite its rich historical contributions to societies everywhere (Ali & Al-Aswad, 2012; Lewis, 2003; Renima, Tiliouine, & Estes, 2016a, 2016b; Tiliouine & Estes, 2016), the region also is one of the world's lesser developed regions and remains a center of socio-political-religious conflict—a complex and enduring conflict that prevents many of its people from moving forward toward shared peace and prosperity (Freedom House, 2018; Fund for Peace, 2018; Imani, 2018). Sadly, thousands of the region's people have become embroiled in these conflicts, at

© Springer Nature Switzerland AG 2019
M. J. Sirgy et al., *Combatting Jihadist Terrorism through Nation-Building*, Human Well-Being Research and Policy Making, https://doi.org/10.1007/978-3-030-17868-0_2

the cost of their own lives and those of others, including foreign nationals (Estes & Sirgy, 2014; SIPRI, 2018).

This chapter explores a series of recurrent questions related to the complex relationships that have and continue to exist between the region's Jews, Christians and Muslims. Before approaching these questions, however, it is important to note the following: (1) diversity-related social conflict is not new to the MENA region–rather it is embedded in centuries of conflict within and between many of these countries, including internal terrorism; (2) the region's conflicts are not strictly religious but many are rooted in centuries-old ethnic divisions that have sparked violence both within and outside of the region[1] (3) fresh water, not petroleum, is, by far, the region's most important and most scarce natural resource as are its highly sought after agricultural, fisheries, carpets and artistic products; and, (4) despite their long history of inter-tribal and intra-regional conflict, the Jewish, Christian, and Islamic peoples of the MENA region have been among the most inventive and poetic people in humanity's history.[2] Simply listening to the singing of the lyrical religious music of any of the three religions is sufficiently powerful to transport one to ever higher levels of personal and collective well-being, even to ecstasy as is witnessed in the rhythmic dances of the Sufi Muslims and Orthodox Jews. The region's extraordinary megalithic architectural genius also cannot be ignored. Who, for example, has not gazed upon the great pyramids or the sphinx on the Giza Plateau and not been transported to another time, space, dimension, or state of being? These wonders of the world are among the region's contributions to humanity that long will survive each of us living today. In the same context, one must show a sense of awe to the seemingly divine-inspired sacred geometry of many of the region's ancient megalithic structures, a geometry that still is not fully understood by contemporary scientists and mathematicians but which clearly are oriented to the stars and movements of planets (Clagett, 1999; Sobhanbredin, 2018).

---

[1]A substantial number of the region's people trace their genetic roots back to ancient Semitic populations; thus, many of the region's Jews, Christians, and Muslims share at least a portion of their genetic material with one another, albeit with measurable regional, cultural, and social exceptions. This is an important fact in that it both contributes to conflict between the various social ethnic groups, as is the case with many families, but also to the increased possibility of eventually promoting peace in the region given the extraordinarily large nature of the extended family relationships that exist between and among the region's peoples (one has to be appreciate even the small bridges that offer the possibility of reducing conflict and promoting peace) (Gibbons, 2000; Wikipedia, 2018a).

[2]The 21 nations of the North African and Middle Eastern region (MENA region) are among the most diverse and conflict-ridden regions in the world. And, yet, the diverse peoples of the region share many DNA and cultural characteristics in common as they do their commitment to monotheism and monotheistic religious practices that date back to God's covenant with Abraham/Ibrahim (אַבְרָהָם/ إِبْرَاهِيم,(*Genesis* 25:7)). The region's conflicts, as described in this chapter, are enmeshed in deeply-rooted diversity-related social conflicts that are more cultural and historical in origin than religious.

This chapter focuses on three major sets of issues pertaining to the region, most of them deeply rooted in its ancient past and the shift from polytheism to monotheism within the context of contemporary patterns of social, political, economic, and technological development, quality of life, and well-being. Among others, the chapter's central goals are:

1. To briefly summarize the rich socio-political-cultural-religious and, as possible, technological history that has shaped the origins of the MENA region and beyond the MENA region to the more than 100 other countries that are predominately Muslim (OIC, 2018).[3]
2. To identify the context through which underlying causes and external drivers of the diversity-related social conflicts that has persisted in the region since virtually the seventh century. And,
3. To lay the foundation for the rich discussions that will be covered in subsequent chapters to help identify a range of peaceful solutions for bringing an end to the conflict, warfare, and terrorism–three conditions that prevent the region's fuller development and the emergence of a *New Islamic Golden Age* in which Jews and Christians are full and equal participants with Muslims.

2.2 Brief History of the Nations and Cultures of the MENA Region

The MENA region has a population of approximately 411 million people or about 23% of 1800 million Muslims worldwide (OIC, 2018). Of significance, too, is that the region includes a disproportionate number of children under the age of 15 years, especially in the predominately Islamic countries of North Africa. Algeria's under 15 years of age cohort, for example, makes up approximately a third to one-half of the country's population (Roudi, 2011).[4] This demographic phenomenon figures prominently in the recurring social conflicts associated with reduced economic opportunities that engulf large expanses of the region (James, 1960). But the region's recurrent civil wars and other intra-country conflicts and, in recent decades, impersonal acts of terrorism impose an even greater burden on the region's peoples to achieve peace. It is a state of peace that generally offers greater opportunities for, accelerated rates of socio-economic-political and technological development, e.g., Afghanistan, Iran, Iraq, Syria, and Yemen. In recent decades, the recurrent social conflicts and reduced economic opportunities are also considered in the context of the creation of the State

---

[3]The *Organization of Islamic Cooperation* (OIC) represents some 1800 million Muslims living in 53 countries with predominately Muslim populations and four nations with substantial but minority concentrations of Muslims (https://www.oic-oci.org/).

[4]Algeria illustrates the disproportionate number of young people living in many of the region's developing countries (see https://www.populationpyramid.net/algeria/2018/). This demographic challenge places enormous demands on the financial and social care resources of families, local communities, and the welfare arrangements at the provincial and national levels.

of Israel by the United Nations in May 1948. That decision led to the displacement of hundreds of thousands of Arab-Palestinians from lands that they, too, regarded as theirs (Lewis, Holt, & Lambton, 1971). As noted earlier, the hope that most of these geographically displaced people would be totally absorbed into the surrounding countries has not come to pass and the resettlement camps have been permanent homes to several generations of some families.

Readers should note, too, that most of the region's post-colonial countries are peaceful and are making substantial progress in providing for the needs of their steadily increasing populations (Estes, 2019; Shaikin & Estes, 2018; SIPRI, 2018; UNDP, 2018; World Bank, 2018). The region's "Gulf States" (e.g., Bahrain, Kuwait, Oman, Qatar, Saudi Arabia and the United Arab Emirates), for example, cooperate with one another in carrying out a broad range of joint financial, shipping, exploration, and water management activities (Tétreault, Okruhlik, & Kapiszewski, 2011). These are remarkable achievements in a region that historically has been characterized by conflicts that consistently have deprived them of the critical resources needed to accelerate the pace of national and subnational development (Tiliouine & Estes, 2016).

The religious and cultural history of the MENA region spans a period of at least 7000, possibly much longer to 11,500 years (Schoch, 1992). The periods ascribed to the great flood that is recorded in virtually all the sacred scriptures worldwide[5] and, today, marks the beginning of new civilizations built on those of the past of which humanity no longer has a memory (Hancock, 2015). Unfortunately, much of the region's history, even after 11,500 BCE, were not recorded except for powerful images on stone carvings of epic stories such as the *Epic of Gilgamesh*, recordings of major war victories (rarely defeats) n stone stele, business transactions recorded on tens of thousands, likely millions, of clay tablets recorded in cuneiform, the majority of which have yet to be interpreted. During the more recent period of dynastic Egypt, wondrous tomb paintings and an abundance of hieroglyphic writings on papyri, and carvings on megalith structures also came into being. All these intellectual and megalithic world treasures speak to the values, norms, traditions, and overarching philosophies that surrounded collective life of the periods reported on. These treasures which, from a macroscopic perspective, provide us with rich insights into the cultures, legal and military systems, as well as the arts of these very ancient societies—whose lives have yet to be fully understood, e.g., again, the "sacred geometry" of the Egyptian pyramids and those that emerged many centuries later in other

---

[5] According to Kerr (2011), the best way to find (the estimate of Biblical events) is to take known historical dates and work backwards from there using dates and durations in the Bible. The Mesha Stele, (for example), has been dated to about 840–850 BCE and seems to clearly describe the time of Omri. If we assume it was written when the events happened, not long afterwards, we can use it to work backwards. Omri's reign began in the 31st year of Asa and lasted twelve years, which means that Asa's reign began around 870–890. Previously, Rehoboam ruled for 17 and Abijah for three. Although the transition is not entirely clear to me, the prior ruler was apparently Solomon for 40 years. In his fourth year, he started to build the temple, which was 480 years after leaving Egypt. So that takes us back 20 + 36 + 480 = 536 years further, to 1406–1426 BCE as the dates for the exodus.

unrelated world regions including the Temple of Angor Wat in Cambodia, the pyramids of mezzo-America, the ancient temples and written scripts of India, among others, that continue to emerge almost each year, e.g., Gokebki Tepe that dates back to well before 11,500 BCE (http://gobeklitepe.info/).

Some of the values of the ancients of this period have been communicated to us have great relevance for the substance of this paper. This knowledge was passed on to us through the few surviving scrolls saved from the destruction of the *Library at Alexandria* (c. 285–c. 246 BCE)[6] and, even more recently, from the collection of widely distributed translations of ancient works in all areas of the sciences, arts, and humanities into Arabic[7] by scholars associated with the *House of Wisdom* in Baghdad (fourth to seventh centuries CE–1258 CE). Sadly, most of the knowledge in these collections was destroyed by Mongol forces who came into the MENA region led by Genghis Khan. The hundreds of thousands of the ancient works that had been translated into Arabic by teams of Muslims, Jews, and Christian scholars working side by side with one another over a period of many centuries held no value to these ancient warriors (Gutas, 1998; Guzman, 1985).

2.2.1 From Polytheism to Monotheism

Monotheism initially spread slowly during the centuries leading up to the first millennium of the modern Era, apart from the teachings of the Pharaoh Akhenaten [c. 1427 BCE–1336 BCE] who succeeded in replacing polytheism, at least for a short period, with monotheism in the form of the Sun God, *Ra* (Dodson, 2009). Akhenaten's establishment of a new capital in Amarna located in Upper Egypt and devoted exclusively to the worship of *Ra* was demolished following his early death, likely at the hands of the high priests who felt undermined by the new religion which excluded a major role for them or for their pantheon of half-human-half-animal gods whose worship they were charged with to preserve.

The Jews were the first Semitic people to introduce monotheism on a systematic basis to own religion and, indirectly, to the religions of non-Jewish peoples with whom they shared their homeland. During their early years as a people whose 12 tribes were organized under a shared set of religious beliefs and cultural practices, the earliest Jews continued to struggle with polytheism as evidenced by the intense anger expressed by Moses toward his people when descending from Mount Sinai with the *Ten Commandments* only to find his people worshiping a "golden calf" (an ancient deity whose origin is in ancient Mesopotamian and the Egyptian cosmology). With

---

[6]The Great Library of Cordoba of the Umayyad Dynasty in Andalusia with its thousands of illuminated manuscripts that survived the sacking of Bagdad was destroyed shortly after 1492 during the Spanish Inquisition when about 500,000 of its priceless translated manuscripts that were either burnt, thrown into rivers, or otherwise destroyed! (Al-Azzawi, 2018).

[7]Other languages were spoken as well but, in the end, everything regard to be value was translated into Arabic, e.g., Farsi, Hebrew, Aramaic, Syriac, Greek and Latin; also, occasionally Sanskrit, which was used to translate the old Indian manuscripts in astronomy and mathematics.

the new revelations from God brought to them by Moses, once understood, however, Jews rapidly abandoned polytheism and accepted *Yahweh* as the one and only true god, a core belief that unites Jews worldwide even today. Though they adopted monotheism, early Jews maintained the retaliatory principles of *lex talionis*, blood sacrifice, as the most appropriate way of making acceptable offerings to God, as well as principles based on love and respect of fellow believers as outlined in the first five books of the *Old Testament* (also referred to as the *Pentateuch*).

Christians and Muslims also adopted monotheism, albeit for many people Christianity's concept of the *Trinity* (God the Father, God the Son, and God the Holy Ghost as a single, indivisible, being), challenged the concept of a single god. Even so, Christians, like the Jews, adopted the principles of the first four "commandments" of the Abrahamic C*ovenant* as the foundation on which the core principles of their own theology rests:

1. *I am the Lord thy God and you shall not have any gods before me*
2. *You shall not make for yourself any idol, nor bow down to it or worship it*
3. *You shall not misuse the name of the Lord your God*
4. *You shall remember and keep the Sabbath day holy*

The remaining six covenants of the Ten Commandments address issues of personal and collective ethical responsibilities between people. These teachings have spanned a period since 3600 BCE to the present.

2.2.2 The Legacy

All three of the *Abrahamic* religions—Judaism, Christianity and, since 632 CE, Islam—developed a strong footing in their geopolitical sub-regions and attracted hundreds of thousands, ultimately millions, of followers over a comparatively brief time. Judaism was the first religion to develop a systematic code of beliefs and placed emphasis on a singular, all powerful, and omniscient god who would accept nothing less than a complete commitment to Him with the requirement that all other deities be put as under. For this reason, the first four of the Ten Commandments handed down by God to Moses on Mount Sinai were to form the basis on which humanity which would shift from polytheism to monotheism.

But believers of all three Abrahamic religions also experienced high levels of political persecution, even martyrdom, for their disavowal of state-promulgated religions. For Christians these persecutions ended in the late fourth and early sixth centuries CE following the conversion of Roman *Emperor Constantine* and his wife the *Empress Helena* to Christianity (Green, 2010). For the first time in their history, Christians were able to engage in public worship in the public as well as to erect churches and sponsor religious schools. They also were appointed to important public positions, own businesses, and to take up arms to fight on behalf of the newly reorganized armies of the period (likely the origin of the unique military competence that is attributed to Israelis in past and contemporary wars).

Muslims, too, often were the targets of state-sponsored persecution. They also experienced widespread martyrdom at the hands of divisional factions within Christianity and others who eventually gained control of the state institutions. These persecutions went back and forth between Christians and Muslims, and Jews for many centuries and, today, as in the past, centered on the acquisition of land, religious relics, and political domination of often distant "holy lands" by alternating majority/minority populations. Muslims also were appointed to important public positions including as government officials and senior military officers. Muslims, instead of focusing on interfaith cooperation, devoted their attention to advances in the arts and architecture, science and technology, translations of ancient texts, and the steady expansion of Islam to new populations across vast expanses of territories not previously exposed to the Prophet's teaching as revealed by God in the *Qur'an* and in subsequent writings prepared by his early disciples (el-Aswad, 2019, this book; Renima, Tiliouine, & Estes, 2016a, 2016b).

2.2.3 The Historical Record of Inter-Religious Conflicts and Socio-Political Development in the Region

Table 2.1, which due to page limitations will not be discussed in detail in this chapter, summarizes the major social, political, and economic events (including major conflicts) that occurred both within the Muslim world following the death of the Prophet. The table also captures events and wars between Muslims, Christians and Jews over the centuries that followed, including conflicts associated the establishment of the State of Israel by the United Nations in 1948 and, with it, the forced displacement of hundreds of thousands of Arab Palestinians from lands that they, too, regarded as their own.

2.3 Judaism, Christianity, and Islam: Shared Beliefs and Origins of Conflict

Despite their often-profound political differences adherents to all three Abrahamic religions shared many values and practices. It is inevitable that they would do so given the cultural heritage that all three groups hold in common with one another, their shared histories of persecution and collective tragedies and to the very large, but mostly resource poor, geographic space that all three groups occupy.[8] Until the modern era when large petroleum reserves were discovered nearly all of its economic activity in the region was based on the harvesting of agricultural and fishery products, metallurgy, the creation of jewelry and hand-made carpets for trade with neighboring

---

[8]The MENA region is about 90% of the size of the contiguous United States, albeit a large portion of the region consists of deserts with very scarce water supplies.

Table 2.1 Historical events in Hebraic, Christian, and Muslim Relations, 12000 BCE–2018 CE

Historical events of the middle and near east

The Ancient Middle and Near East

- 12,000 BCE Small houses in pits developed in regions of Jordan and Syria
- 11,500 BCE the construction of Gobekli Tepe in Turkey—likely the earliest known archeological site in the world. Uncovered in the early twenty-first century by staff of the German Archeological Institute
- 8000 BCE Settlements at Nevali Cori in present-day Turkey established
- 5000 BCE Wheel and plow invented
- 3760 BCE—date of creation according to some interpretations of Jewish chronology
- 3600 BCE—first civilization in the world: Sumer (city-states) in modern-day southern Iraq
- 3500 to 3000 BCE—one of the first appearances of wheeled vehicles in Mesopotamia
- 3500 BCE—beginning of desertification of the Sahara: the shift from a habitable region to a barren desert
- 3500 BCE—first cities in Egypt
- 3300 BCE—earliest hieroglyphs
- 3100 BCE Cuneiform writing invented
- 3100 BCE—King Narmer unifies the Upper and Lower Egyptian Kingdoms, in Egypt and gives birth to the world's first nation
- 3000 BCE Bronze Age begins
- 3000 BCE—first examples of Sumerian writing in Mesopotamia, in the cities of Uruk and Susa (cuneiform writings)
- 1867 BCE Babylon founded by Amorite dynasty
- 1600–1360 BCE Egypt dominates the region of Canaan and Syria
- 1250 BCE Hebrews establish a kingdom in Palestine
- 1200–1050 BCE Collapse of the Bronze Age. Within a period of forty to fifty years at the end of the thirteenth and the beginning of the twelfth century almost every significant city in the eastern Mediterranean world was destroyed, many of them never to be occupied again (Drews, 1995)
- 1041 BCE Jerusalem designated the capital of the Kingdom of Israel
- 1000 BCE Iron Age begins
- 600 BCE Babylon conquered; Cyrus the Great creates the Persian Empire
- 331 BCE Alexander the Great overpowers Persia; bloody warfare ensues

The Middle and Near East at the Start of a New Millennium

- 50 CE Christianity emerges
- 5th–15th—a thousand years of the European Dark Ages
- 632 CE Death of the Prophet in Medina (Saudi Arabia)
- 634 CE Series of Muslim conquests begin; Arab empire founded
- 711–788—The Umayyad conquest of Hispania; the conquest resulted in the establishment of the independent Emirate of Córdoba
- 759–1258 Baghdad becomes capital of Arab-Islamic empire
- 1095–1291—the Christian Crusades with the goal of returning control of the Holy Lands from Islamic control
- 1200 Mongols invade the Middle East ending the Arab-Islamic empire
- 1491 Granada surrenders and relinquishes the last Muslim-controlled city on the Iberian Peninsula to the expanding Crown of Castile via the *Treaty of Granada*
- 1517–1918 Ottoman Empire extends through most of the Arab world

(continued)

Table 2.1 (continued)

Historical events of the middle and near east

1900s

- 1901 Oil discovered in Iran
- 1914 World War I begins, Ottomans align with Germany
- 1918 World War I ends; Britain and France occupy much of the Middle East after the collapse of the Ottoman Empire
- 1919–1921 Franco-Syrian War; Syria divided into two mandates: French Mandate of Syria and Lebanon and the British mandate of Palestine
- 1921 Faisal becomes King of Iraq 1922 The dissolution of the Ottoman Empire (1908–1922) began with the *Second Constitutional Era* with the *Young Turk Revolution*. It restored the *Ottoman Constitution of 1876* and brought in multi-party politics with a two stage electoral system (electoral law) under the Ottoman parliament
- 1922 European power divide up major territories of the previous Ottoman Empire as their own colonies
- 1923 *Treaty of Lausanne* secured international recognition for the new Turkish state which was formally declared on 29 October
- 1932 Kingdom of Saudi Arabia founded
- 1933–1936 Assyrians in Simele are massacred by Iraqi armed forces
- 1934 Saudi-Yemeni War
- 1935 Persia becomes Iran
- 1936 Jewish immigration to Palestine increases
- 1939 World War II begins
- 1939 Britain issues the White Paper limiting the number of Jewish immigrants into Palestine
- 1941 British forces overthrow Iraqi government and install pro-British leaders
- 1945 World War II ends; the League of Arab States founded
- 1946 Jordan, Lebanon and Syria gain independence from Britain and France
- 1946 Terrorists bomb the King David Hotel in Jerusalem, 91 killed
- 1947 Zionist leaders declare war on British in Palestine to get the 1939 White Paper cancelled
- 1947 UN proposes to divide Palestine into an Arab and Jewish state
- 1948 Britain withdraws forces from Palestine
- 1948 Arab-Israeli war develops after Israel declares independence
- 1950 West Bank annexed by Jordan
- 1951 Libya receives independence
- 1952 Hussein Ibn Talal declared King of Jordan
- 1954 Sudan becomes an officially recognized independent republic
- 1956 Jordan and Israel establish a truce
- 1958 Abdul-Karim overthrows Iraq monarch and prime minister
- 1959 Oil is discovered in Libya
- 1961 First Kurdish-Iraq War erupts in Iraq
- 1967 Israel occupies Sinai, Golan heights, West Bank and Gaza during Six-Day War
- 1975–1990 Lebanese Civil War prevails
- 1976 Syria invades Lebanon
- 1979 Saddam Hussein becomes president of Iraq
- 1980–1989 Iran-Iraq War rages, casualties' range in the millions
- 1982 Israel invades Lebanon to drive out PLO
- 1990 North and South Yemen merge into the Republic of Yemen
- 1990 Iraq invades Kuwait
- 1991 The Gulf War begins in response to Iraq's invasion of Kuwait
- 1993 Oslo I agreement signed setting up Israeli-Palestinian Peace settlement
- 1995 Palestine granted full control of part of West Bank and Gaza after Oslo II agreement signed
- 1995 Israeli Prime Minister, Yitzhak Rabin assassinated
- 1998 Taliban inches closer to power in Kabul after a series of military victories

(continued)

Table 2.1 (continued)

Historical events of the middle and near east

2000s
- 2000 Israeli troops vacate Lebanon
- 2001 Destruction of Trade Towers in New York by Terrorists from the Middle East region
- 2003 The US, United Kingdom, Australia and Poland invade Iraq; Sadam Hussein removed from power
- 2001—Members of al-Qaeda attacked sites in the U.S.
- 2003—The 2003 Iraq War
- 2004 to present—Shia insurgency in Yemen
- 2005 Syrian troops leave Lebanon as a result of the Cedar Revolution
- 2006 The 2006 Israel-Lebanon conflict; Saddam Hussein executed for "crimes against humanity"
- 2010 Arab Spring, which culminates in the Syrian Civil War with involvement of many regional powers to either support the Syrian opposition or the ruling Ba'ath party
- 2011–2012 Syrian uprising; thousands of citizens protest for the overthrow of the government; widespread marches, hunger strikes, rioting, and vandalism 2000—Israeli troops leave Lebanon
- 2014 ISIS rises in Iraq and Syria; Rival groups try to overthrow Syrian president
- 2015 Russia carries out its first air strikes in Syria, saying they target the Islamic State group, but the West and Syrian assert that they target anti-Assad rebels
- 2016 Syria in a virtual state of political collapse associated with its long-lasting civil war
- 2017–2018 American-led coalition wars in Iraq and Afghanistan pass the 10-year mark with a legacy of large numbers of casualties within residents of the targeted countries and the multinational coalition forces

Adapted from World Atlas (2016)

This table was last updated by the World Atlas on September 19, 2016 and supplemented by the author using a variety of historical data sources in October 2018 (mostly the *CIA Factbook*, 2018, *Encyclopedia Britannica On Line*, 2017; the writings of Lewis, 2003, 2017; and various on-line historical sites).

countries, as well as the region's skilled artists who converted its abundant deposits of sand into delicate glass creations, magnificent hand painted tiles, and pottery (clay and glass) that adorn the homes of the well-off worldwide.

Harmony and peace in the region, two necessary prerequisites for achieving high levels of quality of life and well-being, were interrupted repeatedly by disputes over territorial boundaries and its scarce natural and human resources (Krieger, 2016). Not infrequently, direct attacks initiated by powerful elites against less powerful states and tribal groups also has been widespread in the region (Table 2.1). Attacks from outside the region continue to be frequent, especially from nations seeking to make claim on the region's lands, its temples and shrines and, over the last 100 years or so, on its important oil resources. Internally to the MENA region there have been recurrent civil wars, a recent and highly influential "Arab Spring" (that, to date, has not achieved its promise), and decades-old revolutionary movements in Afghanistan, Iran, Iraq, and Syria. Each of these movements' goals have, in one way or another, sought to restore the region's people to their former glory experienced centuries ago during the *Islamic Golden Age* (Estes & Sirgy, 2014). The region also is engaged in recurrent struggles that seek to establish a renewed global Caliphate (Estes & Tiliouine, 2016) and to return all its countries to Shari'a law (Keshavjee, 2016). None of these struggles are entirely new since they reflect challenges that have confronted the region's people and their governments since well before the birth of the Prophet and the early formative years of Islam (Renima, Tiliouine, & Estes, 2016a).

In the section that follows we will attempt to sort out the historical drivers that may have influenced contemporary conflicts occurring within the MENA region and beyond the MENA region to other areas of the world.[9] As noted, the current chapter focuses on the long expanse of the histories of the Jews, Christians and Islamic peoples in the region and their interaction with one another—both peaceful (see Box 2.1) and conflictual (see Box 2.2). We use this dialogue to highlight the shared socio-cultural, economic, biological and, to a lesser extent the political systems that have historically characterized the region and are the basis of current thoughts and behaviors in the regions peoples. For example, the continuing emphasis on an "eye for an eye" dictum that persists in all three of the region's major religions. We will also briefly summarize the major social challenges that have confronted the region's people in their efforts to live together in harmony.

Box 2.1: Amadiya, Iraq: Fertile Harmony for Christians, Muslims, and Jews

Amadiya has held a space in the now semiautonomous province of Kurdistan, Iraq for centuries. It sits on a mesa with two mountain ranges as its guardians throughout history. While the recent history has included crackdowns on the village by Saddam Hussein during his regime and the battles with ISIS. There has, however, been a singular constant for the village over the religious tolerance. That is religious tolerance between its Muslims, Christians, and Jews. At the center of that tolerance is the Jewish holy figure Hazana. Now a village of about 9000 people, the clear majority of whom are Sunni Muslim Kurds, the historic diverse populations, until the early twentieth Century, was made up of approximately equally distributed faiths of Muslim, Christian, and Jews. The village enjoyed 10 mosques, two churches, and two synagogues. There are still about 30 families of Christians in the village, the Jews had all left for Israel after 1948. Jewish pilgrims and tourists are still welcome in the village. The reverence for Hazana, a prophet of unknown antiquity, has kept the respect and tolerance for the three Abrahamic religions alive in a time when tolerance in the region has been seriously wanting. His tomb is in Amadiya and all three religions go to his tomb to pray. Hazana is thought to offer fertility to supplicants. The villagers find religious tolerance as completely normal and say it has been taught to them by their parents, whose parents taught it to them, and so on back through the centuries. A veteran of the Kurdish pesh merga Special

---

[9]The Tigris-Euphrates River Valley and the Fertile Crescent (River Valley Civilization Guide, 2017). Mesopotamia is an area geographically located between the Tigris and Euphrates rivers. Mesopotamia means the land between two rivers. Mesopotamia began as urban societies in southern Iraq in 5000 BC and ends in the 6th century BCE. The exact location of the two "missing" rivers of the four referred to in the Old Testament is not currently known, albeit using Google Earth their probable dried up river beds have been approximated.

Forces, who is now a caretake at the Chaldean church says. "That's the beauty of Amadiya. In this small place you can find Muslims, Jews, Christians."
   Adapted from: Norland (2017).

Box 2.2: Post Arab Spring: Islamist Spill-Over Heightens Tensions Between Christians and Muslims
There was a great deal of hope and joy in the casting off the bonds of several authoritarian regimes in what has become known as the Arab Spring. People celebrated in the streets of several capitals in the Mideast region with the hope that these populist movements would bring a better quality of life to the people in the region. There was hope on the streets of Cairo that better days were ahead for all Egyptians, regardless of their faith and political vent. Unfortunately, that has not been the case. Indeed, events that gave birth to an elected Islamist government, and its subsequent removal by the military, has not facilitated an environment of religious harmony, or even enhanced tolerance, among the population of Egypt which includes people of many faiths. There has been a rise in intolerance and violence between Muslims and the Christian (mostly Coptic) minority who make up about 10% of the population of 94 million. Egypt is, by law, an Islamic country, but religious freedom is enshrined in its constitution. It also has had a history of restricting Christians in the practice of their faith. In general, there was support among the Christian minority for the military coup that led to President Abdel Fatah al-Sissi's government. There had been hope among the Christians that Sissi's government would protect them after toppling the Islamists. That has not often been the case. In the post-coup environment there has been a significant increase in attacks on the Christian minority. It is also noted that in the days following the coup, there were a targeted series of attacks on Christians driven by the idea that they were in league with the coup leaders. It is also noted that the continued rise in attacks on Christians are being driven by a rising, and deepening, mistrust between Christians and Muslims. It seems that violence is no longer something that is a rare occurrence. Community leaders report that it can be almost any sort of problem or disagreement between Muslim and Christian neighbors that may well turn violent and even deadly. Rumors quickly are acted on whether confirmed or not, leading to such things as the burning of homes of Christians on a rumor that these homes were going to be turned into churches. Before the revolution, Christians were targeted mostly by militant groups. The violence has spread with Muslim and Christian citizens turning against each other.
   Adapted from: Raghavan (2016).

This region is home to the world's first urban civilizations (those of Sumer and Ur) in the valley of the Tigris and Euphrates rivers–as well as the two additional historical rivers that are identified in the bible but whose precise location can no longer be identified (River Valley Civilizations, 2017). Obviously, this region's civilizations, have an incredibly rich history which gave humanity its first alphabets (including Cuneiform[10] and the hieroglyphics of dynastic Egypt), ways of measuring time that continue even into the modern era (ancient Sumer and its related cultures of Mesopotamia), our first calendar including the zodiac, the first organized systems of religious beliefs (best expressed through the ancient's Egyptian polytheism but, in time, its adoption of monotheism), its first system of integrated laws that asserted that no man was above the law (ancient Babylonia, including the only rediscovered stone stela on which had been chiseled including the foundational *Code of Hammurabi*) (Hammurabi & King, 2015). These stelae and others also contained an incredibly rich array of teachings (Remina, Tiliouine, & Estes, 2016a, 2016b).

2.4 Abraham and the Emergence of Judaism, Christianity, and Islam (2500 BCE–500 CE)

Abraham (*Arabic: Ibrahim*) was the first and most influential of the ancient prophets and spiritual leaders that guided the world toward monotheism.[11] Estimated to have lived for nearly two centuries,[12] Abraham introduced the region's peoples to monotheism, an idea that proved initially difficult for even the most progressive teachers of them to accept. This was especially difficult given the panoply of deities that made up the panoply of gods associated with the natural environment and the recurrent cycles of life associated with humans, flora, and fauna. With Abraham, however, the monotheistic teachings concerning God were straightforward and readily understandable by most of the population, i.e., *I am God, the only God and, through me, comes all life and that on which life depends* (Hicks & Hicks, 2007).

---

[10]Cuneiform was the first written language and developed in Mesopotamia. It is distinguished by its wedge-shaped marks on clay tablets (made by means of a blunt reed for a stylus). This communication system was created by the ancients Sumerians between the years 5000 BCE and 4000 BCE and was the world's first known written language. Cuneiform writing was so influential that it spread throughout successor civilizations following the fall of Sumer in the 1st century CE (Bertman, 2005).

[11]The Egyptian Pharaoh Akhenaten also briefly brought a brief, but dramatic, end to polytheism from throughout his Empire during the fourteenth century BCE and, in its place, established a theocracy devoted to the Sun god, *Ra*, based on monotheism. The Pharaoh built an entire city, Amarna, devoted to the Sun god from which all polytheistic idols and practices were banned (Charles River Editors & Carabas, 2018).

[12]This is an especially remarkable achievement given that most of the people of the period rarely lived longer than 40 years on average—a reality associated with a combination of high rates of infant and child mortality, maternal morbidity, deaths associates with warfare, and generally poor sanitation and health for population-as-a-group (Liljas, 2015).

The ancient Jews quickly adopted this belief system and, as directed by God through Abraham, desisted in their polytheistic practices (Gordon, 1966).

Abraham is not only considered to be the founder of Judaism but also the transformational prophet whose written and oral teachings shaped early Christianity and Islamic teachings (Khan, 2018). His long life, central role in the ancient religions and the attributed special relationship that is believed to have existed between him and God appreciably enhanced his stature among the region's earliest peoples. The *Dome of the Rock* in Jerusalem (*Qubbat al-Ṣakhrah*),[13] Islam's third holiest site, enshrines the rock on which Abraham's son, Isaac, was to be sacrificed but, in the end, was saved from this blood sacrifice by God's last-minute intercession to Abraham to stop the sacrifice in acknowledgement of Abraham's unwavering obedience to the will of God (*Genesis* 22:1–14).

The relationship between God, Abraham, and others that were to become his chosen people, even during the earliest years of monotheism, was characterized by violence associated with competing tribes of believers and non-believers, those that made legitimate claims on the lands they occupied, as well as with invading tribes of warriors that sought the same land and scarce resources for themselves. Even with the existence of a single, solitary, all powerful God, violence and conflict has remained a constant feature of the peoples of the Middle East and beyond from the earlier dates of recorded history. Nonetheless, Abraham and his successors, laid the foundation for monotheism throughout the then known Western world.

2.5 The Rapid Rise of Judaism (C. 3600 BCE–Present)

As the name implies, Judaism was concentrated among the Jews and related Semitic peoples of North Africa and West Asia who quickly adopted the revelations made to them by God through his prophet Moses during the period of the Exodus from Egypt. These revelations were granted to the already aged Moses following his ascent of Mount Sinai (the precise location of which continues to prove elusive). In exchanges the designation of the Jews for special status among God's people, the revelations were encoded on two stone tablets which are believed to still be housed in the *Ark of the Covenant*, whose whereabouts also continues to elude discovery (but whose location many believe to be in the ancient church of Saint Mary of Zion located in Axum, Ethiopia).

---

[13]*The Dome of the Rock* is located on a rocky outcrop known as Mount Moriah, where, according to Jewish belief, Abraham offered his son Isaac as a sacrifice. The inscriptions inside the building glorify Islam as the final true revelation and culmination of the faiths of Judaism and Christianity.

For adherence to the demanding challenges of the "Ten Commandments," often referred to as the "Mosaic Covenant," the Jews were granted access to "the Promised Lands" in perpetuity—which spanned from … from the Wadi of Egypt to the great river, the Euphrates–the ancestral homelands of land of the Kenites, Kenizzites, Kadmonites (*Genesis 15:18-19; Exodus 19:1-34:30*).[14] All these promises made by God to the Hebrews were to be realized following the Jew's 40-years of wandering in the deserts of the region, a journey that prove too demanding for the already aged Moses to survive. The promises, however, set into motion the displacement of populations from other ancient lands from lands that they, too, considered their own.

The precise dates of the Exodus are unknown but *Kings 6:1* place the event around about 480 years before the construction of Solomon's (First) Temple, implying an exodus beginning at about 1450 BCE—but the date is likely more hypothetical rather than historical, representing a symbolic twelve generations of forty (Plaut & Bamberger, 1981). Of interest, too, is that the population of adult male Jews, whose numbers were closely counted by Hebraic and Roman political authorities, was approximately 600,000 in addition to approximately equal numbers of women and children (*Exodus* 12:37–38).

The Jews eventually settled in their new homeland centered in and around Canaan which, today, in its larger geographical meaning, is known as Palestine and, since 1948, Israel. Religion, along with elaborate religious practices, permeated all aspects of Jewish collective life which centered on the worship of a single God, *Yahweh*. Life for the Jews, even during these early centuries of development, was far from peaceful and was characterized by repeated conflicts associated with their Babylonian exile (538 BCE–70 CE) and those of the steadily expanding Roman Empire that already laid claim to much of the land of the Middle and Near as well as West Asia (230 BCE–400 CE). Jews often were subject to forced labor, indentured servitude, murdered as public sacrifices in Roman circuses and colosseums and, not infrequently, died because of the deeply ingrained feelings of anti-Semitism that existed at the time.

Today, Jews number approximately 14.6 million worldwide, approximately 6.5 million of whom live in Israel and 5.7 million live in the United States—together 84% of the world's total Jewish population. Religious freedom combined with the opportunity to flourish as a people is a hallmark of the Jewish populations of both countries. Jews around the world, especially the large population in USA, have a deep seeded connection to the Holy Land and the historic Jewish presence in the Holy Land.

---

[14] According to *Genesis* 15:18 and *Joshua* 1:4, the land God gave to Israel included everything from the Nile River in Egypt to Lebanon (south to north) and everything from the Mediterranean Sea to the Euphrates River (west to east). So, what land has God stated belongs to Israel? All the land modern Israel currently possesses, plus all the land of the Palestinians (the West Bank and Gaza), plus some of Egypt and Syria, plus all of Jordan, plus some of Saudi Arabia and Iraq. Israel currently possesses only a fraction of the land God has promised. See, too, https://www.gotquestions.org/Israel-land.html.

2.6   The Rapid Growth of Christianity (50 CE–Present)

And, then, there are the Christians (50 CE–present). The "historical Jesus," the central figure of Christianity, is believed to have been born in Nazareth to a teenage Jewish woman aged 15–16 years old and to a much older Jewish stepfather, Joseph, a carpenter, sometime between 6 BCE and 4 BCE (Meier, 1991). Jesus is believed by Christians to have resulted from a "virgin birth."[15] His conception is believed to have resulted from the divine intervention of God in the form of the Holy Ghost. Further, Mary's virginity is believed to have been restored following the birth of Jesus, thus, her virginity remained intact despite having given birth to Jesus.

Jesus did not reveal himself to be "The Christ" (the anointed one) or as "God made man"[16] until much later in his human manifestation and likely not before beginning his public ministry at or about age 30, though, the *New Testament* teaches that his deity was already known to Mary. The proofs that followed Jesus' public ministry confirmed what already were the signs of the arrival of the Messiah through his performance of the expected biblical miracles (including restoring sight to the blind and rising from the dead), insightful teachings well beyond his age and level of formal spiritual education, the ability to gather a large number of followers, and his willingness to be sacrificed as a martyr who, through his death, would absorb all "the sins of the world" (*Luke* 1:26-38).

Little is known about the early life of Jesus until he began his public ministry and what we do know was not written until many decades following his death at about the age of 33. Jesus as "The Christ" was not known until quite late in his public life and was lamented by the early group of men who joined him as apostles. Especially troublesome early on was Jesus proclaiming himself to be the "Son of God", thereby, suggesting a separate identity from that of the Father. Similarly, Jesus co-equal identity as the Holy Ghost also proved to be problematic to many since an identity as the Father, Son, and Holy Ghost bordered on polytheism and required several councils of the Roman church to resolve and, then, based on faith rather than objective evidence.[17]

---

[15]The virgin birth of Jesus is the belief that Jesus was conceived in the womb of his mother Mary through the Holy Spirit without the agency of a human father and born while Mary was still a virgin. The *New Testament* references are Matthew 1:18-25 and Luke 1:26-38; it is not expressly mentioned elsewhere in the Christian scriptures and many modern scholars believe there exists very little scientific evidence to support such a widespread belief, albeit it is taken by most Christians as an article of faith and no one subject to objective proof or rejection. This belief is central to Christianity inasmuch as God could not results from the sexual union of human man and a human woman.

[16]In Christianity, Christ (Greek: Χριστός, Christós, meaning "the anointed one") is a title for the savior and redeemer who would bring salvation to the whole House of Israel. Christians believe Jesus is the Israelite messiah foretold in both the Hebrew Bible and the Christian Old Testament.

[17]The Trinitarian Christian doctrine holds that God is one God, but three coeternal consubstantial persons or hypostases—the Father, the Son (Jesus Christ), and the Holy Spirit—as "one God in three Divine Persons" (Hillar, 2012).

In any case, as the son of Jewish parents, raised as a Jew in a Jewish culture, Jesus very strongly identified himself as a Jew … as did all his initial followers/leaders except for the Roman Paul (known in his early life as Saul). Though a fervent practitioner of Judaism and with a deep knowledge of the teaching of the *Old Testament* disavowed the philosophy of an "eye for an eye" (also referred to as *lex talionis,* or "the law of retaliation") that permeated most of the regions religious and philosophical systems (Encyclopedia Britannica, 2018). The basic tenets of the "eye for an eye" philosophy and was chiseled into a remarkable stela that has permanently summarized the "Code of Hammurabi" which give civilization its first system of integrated laws (Hammurabi & King, 2015). The laws that formed the code were deeply tied to the principle of *lex talionis* and specified precise punishments for classes or groups of crimes.

Jesus, bringing with him, even as a young man, a "new testament" taught his followers that the unforgiving, often brutal, nature of the practices associated its enforcement, emphasized the centrality of forgiveness by self and others was the new covenant between God and man. Similarly, Jesus taught that blood sacrifice no longer would be required of those who sought to live their lives consistent with God's desires; instead, charity (love) toward others should guide religiously-based practices. Ironically, of course, Jesus Himself, in proclaiming Himself as "The Christ" and the conveyer of a new covenant between God and man became a victim of both the retaliatory behavior of the type promoted by *lex talionis* as well as of a blood sacrifice—His own brutal death through Crucifixion.

The death of Jesus associated with both sets of then prevailing practices marked the beginning of the first millennium of the Common Era (the era before the birth of Jesus Christ) and created a major religious rift between the first Christians and the Jewish religious leaders whom the early Christians blamed for advancing Christ's death by Roman civil authorities, but at the urging of Jewish religious authorities (Levine, 2009; Wilken, 2003). The Roman Church in recent years separated itself from such an assertion and, instead, places the responsibility for the death of Jesus directly in the hands of the Romans who responded to Christ's death as being associated the mob mentality of the time—consisting of not only Jews, but Romans, and the many idolaters who populated Imperial Rome of the period.

Christianity emerged out of the shadows of Roman society to emerge as a socially recognized (and marginally acceptable) religion through actions taken by the late to adopt *Christianity Emperor Constantine the Great* (272 CE–337 CE) (Gill, 2018).[18] Following the integration of Christians into Roman society, Jews and Christians lived side by side with one another and, indeed, most of the early Christians, including the 12 apostles and Jesus himself, were religious Jews. In due course, many Romans eventually joined with the early Christians in their acceptance of Jesus as God, but this required several generations to accomplish. All, though, eventually were persecuted by the Roman rulers of the period and were stigmatized frequently by the

---

[18]The first state-sponsored persecution of Christians by the Roman government took place under the emperor Nero in 64 CE after the *Great Fire of Rome*. With the passage in 313 AD of the *Edict of Milan*, persecution of Christians by the Roman state ceased.

Romans with whom they shared communal life. The latter was highly problematic and forced the blended group of Jewish and Roman Christians to separate themselves from the middle mass of Roman society. Instead, they took their religious services underground, often in caves and tunnels located not far from the catacombs of the hill on which the Vatican was eventually to be constructed. The Vatican itself is at the apex of an ancient Christian cemetery, many of whom perished as martyrs in the coliseums of Rome. It was not until the assumption of imperial power by the Emperor Constantine that Christians were permitted to self-identify themselves as such and, of course, to build dedicated religious shrines, temples, and churches. The legacy of centuries-long persecution by intolerant religious groups, though, was not soon forgotten by the Christians and, even given their teachings of tolerance and love for evil-doers, informed their future relationships with other groups including, in time, both Jews and Muslims.

The (Protestant) *Reformation* was spearheaded by Martin Luther of Germany (1483–1546).[19] The *Reformation* upended the primacy of the Roman Church and Papal authority (Pope Leo X in 1520) in political, military, religious and all other communal matters throughout Europe. This schism provoked a high level of violence in on the continent, including major persecutions of Catholics and Protestants. In England, the establishment of the Anglican church with the monarch, rather than the Pope, emerged as the church's secular leader on earth. The horrendous struggles between Queen Elizabeth I and Mary, Queen of Scots, led to the beheading of Queen Mary and the designation of Mary's cousin, Queen Elizabeth I, as the head of the Anglican Church in England, Scotland and, in time, Wales and what was to become Northern Ireland in the twentieth century. Though comparatively peaceful today, the problems of religious intolerance continue to manifest themselves in selected areas of Great Britain between Catholics and Protestants, Jews and, given their rapidly increasing number as a share of the total population, between these two groups and Muslims. The same pattern permeates much of both the past and contemporary continental Europe (Kaplan, 2007).

The *European Age of Enlightenment* began in the seventeenth century[20] reawakened Greater Europe and the rest of the Western world to a new beginning of scientific and technological development that continues at a dramatic pace even to the present (Gottlieb, 2017). The *Enlightenment* further brought about a separation between the Roman Church and states and, in doing so, permitted people personal self-awareness and reexamination of the role of the Roman church over the personal lives' individuals. The *Enlightenment* also solidified the protestant *Reformation* and allowed many other sects of Protestantism to come into being. All the movements led to a

---

[19]The Reformation was a schism in Western Christianity initiated by Martin Luther and continued by Huldrych Zwingli, John Calvin and other Protestant Reformers in sixteenth and seventeenth century Europe.

[20]A European intellectual movement of the late seventeenth and eighteenth centuries emphasizing reason and individualism rather than tradition. It was heavily influenced by seventeenth-century philosophers such as Descartes, Locke, and Newton, and its prominent exponents include Kant, Goethe, Voltaire, Rousseau, and Adam Smith.

high level of religious diversity within Christianity and permitted the resolution of conflicts within the Church that had been ongoing for nearly a millennium.

2.7 The Rapid Growth of Islam (632 CE–Present)

Islam is the world's most rapidly growing religion and, today, numbers more than 1800 million adherent location in all regions of the world (OIC, 2018). Muslims in the MENA region account for somewhat less than 15% of Muslims worldwide despite the media's preoccupation with the region's major political events, development challenges, and both natural and financial resources that play a disproportionate role in world affairs. The expectation is that Islam will number more than 2000 million followers, possibly the world's largest religion, by the middle of the current century.

In the past, Islam's growth has been associated with its geographic expansion into new lands and territories. Many of the conversions into the religion, at least during its first three centuries, were coerced with the choice given to idolaters and "pagans" of either death or conversion to Islam (Religion of Peace, 2018; Wikipedia, 2018b). Christians used the same approach to Muslims in lands that Christians conquered including the Holy Lands in the Near East (especially in Istanbul, Jerusalem, and in colonized countries of North Africa and the Near East). Only Jews did not proselytize or force conversions to Judaism of the lands they colonized. This latter practice was cultural in origin and stemmed from the belief on the part of Jews, not others, that they were God's "chosen people" and, therefore, forced conversions to Judaism would not have been appropriate.

Among other reasons, Islam's appeal to the masses were based on the richness and straightforward in their presentation of the Islam's core teachings. Figure 2.1 provides a graphical summary of the Islam's major articles of faith. These six articles of faith are easily taught and, in turn, easily understood and internalized. They have proven to be timelessness in their message and embrace all people of other faith traditions. They also are at a level that Islam's articles of faith can readily be substituted for those of other religions (Fig. 2.1).

In addition to Islam's six foundational articles of faith, it also teaches *Five Pillars* of social conduct around which all Muslims must organize their lives. These Pillars of core Islamic religious practice are summarized in Fig. 2.2 and, again, presents the Pillars of ethical conducts are presented in graphical format. All five are equally important although Islam recognizes that many followers for reasons of health, finances, distance and other factors may not be able to undertake the journey (which for many may involve as many as 5000–10,000 miles).

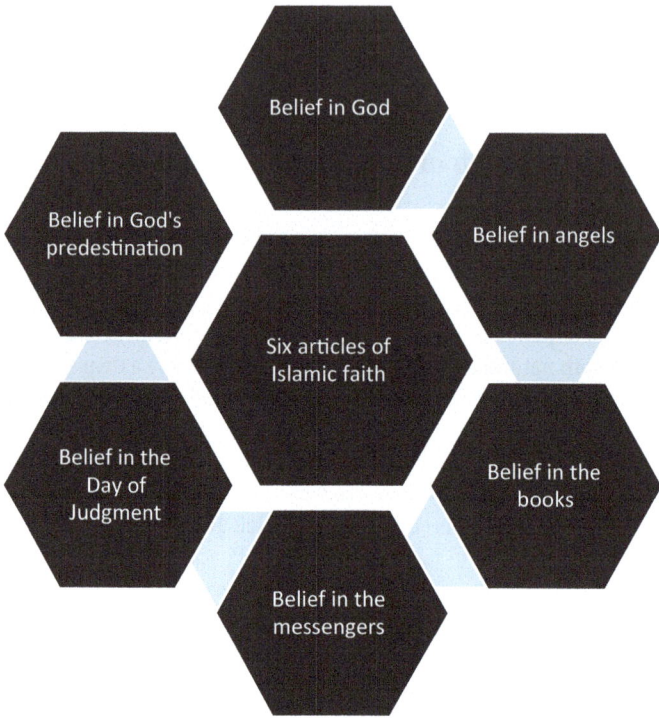

Fig. 2.1 Basic religious articles of Islam. *Source* Adapted from https://commons.wikimedia.org/wiki/File:Six_articles_of_the_Islamic_faith.svg

Fig. 2.2 The five pillars of Islam. *Source* Adapted from https://upload.wikimedia.org/wikipedia/commons/e/ef/Five_pillars_of_Islam.svg

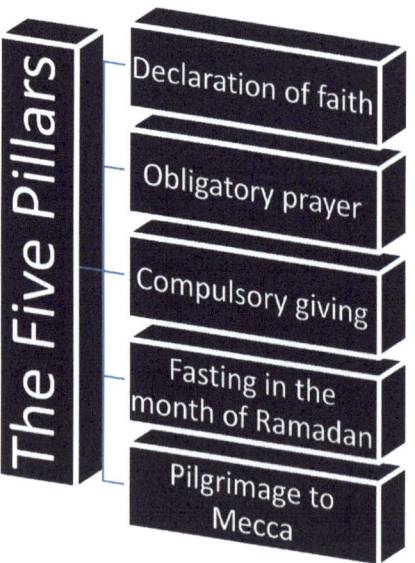

2.7.1 Violence and Islam

There are no teachings in Islam that condone violence; indeed, Islam, like Christianity, is a religion based on love, forgiveness and inclusiveness. The violence associated with Islam is cultural in nature rather than religious. The cultural elements that promote violence are those already identified in the chapter and include those associated with the "eye for an eye" philosophy (*lex talionis*) that originate from the ancient cultures of the Mesopotamia River Valley. Practices such as beheading, torture, the grotesque removal of limbs, the stoning and killing of women for deeds that would not be punishable throughout much of the modern world can be found in the prescribed punishments prescribed for comparable acts identified in the *Code of Hammurabi* and in other legalistic documents by even more ancient history that neither knew nor taught the forgiveness values of Islam or any other of its core values (Hammurabi & King, 2015).

Islam, however, and as summarized in Table 2.1 has a long history of internal and external warfare, occupation, and conflict both with its three major sects and with other religions—*Sunni's* c. 84%, *Shia* c. 10%, and the mystical sect, the *Sufis* c. 6%. Confrontations with the Jews have been on-going with Muslims since the dissolution of the *House of Wisdom* to the establishment of the State of Israel by the United Nations in retribution for the European Jewish holocaust, to the present with Israel's refusal to grant a two-state solution to Israel contemporary political structure. Islam–Christian conflicts predate the decades of the Crusades and has continued well into the present given the high level of socio-political-economic and technological achievements accomplished scholars and scientists associated with the *House of Wisdom* that substantially exceeded those of predominately Christian Protestant countries of Europe and elsewhere (CIA, 2018). These conflicts also are related to the historic seizure of major Christian sites in the *Holy Lands* located in the Near East and Central Asia by Muslims who claimed the right to occupancy despite centuries of earlier occupation of these sites by Christians (Lewis, Holt & Lambton, 1971).

Today, most Islamist Jihad terrorist strikes are directed against Western countries that consist primarily of Christian Protestants and are directed at anonymous citizens located in their capital cities, financial centers, and other centers of political power. Acts of terrorism occur using various modes of transportation, satchel bombs and, in recent years, poisonous substances delivered by either regular or express mail. This terrorism has taken the lives of many totally innocent people over the past two decades and the pattern continues to increase despite hundreds of millions of dollars being spent annually on their containment (START, 2018).

As reported throughout this book the ages of terrorists have become younger and include both young men and women, many of who do not foresee a positive future for themselves over the near term. Terrorists also tend to be repeat offenders and, as suggested above, are motivated by fringe radical clerics or personal interpretations of religious principles despite the teachings of the Islamic religion against suicide and violence toward others. Indeed, most terrorists believe that they will be richly rewarded in an afterlife if their deaths are associated with acts of violence toward non-believers, even idolaters.

2.8   Discussion and Conclusion

The contemporary world is confronting a broad range of diversity-related social conflicts. Many of these are grounded in contrarian religious perspectives and contain remnants of ancient cultures that still affect our behavior and well-being. Many of these conflicts are rooted in especially intransigent geo-political histories and, since the reestablishment of the State of Israel by the United Nations in 1948, conflicts between Arabs and Israelis living together in the MENA region. The displacement of hundreds of thousands of Palestinian Arabs into cities along the West Bank and in specially designed refugee camps, has proven to be an intractable problem especially given its rejection of a workable two-state solution to the perceived injustices experienced by Arab Palestinians.

Central to the region's ancient and contemporary histories and the many factors that function as drivers of the region's quality of life and well is the pace of social development that is taking place both within and outside the region. Especially central to this part of the discussion is that the pace of human progress associated with social, political, economic, technological and even religious development. As already discussed, members of the three Abrahamic religions focused on in this chapter have highly uneven patterns of development, especially among the group of Islamic nations which continue to struggle between tradition and modernization. These challenges also confront the orthodox branches of Judaism and Christianity, most of which are guided by traditional belief systems that prevent these sects from moving fully into the modern era. Islamist Jihad and the embracing of terrorism are closely linked to orthodox branches of their religions and, as a result, are characterized by lower, on average, levels of social development. Lower average levels of quality of life characterize a substantial number of the region's nations, especially those located in the North Africa and West Asia. Orthodoxy, rejection of modernity, and disparity in economic and social well-being present in these nations create a ripe environment for exploitation by those in search of political power and influence.

The remaining chapters of the book focus in depth on the challenges that are confronting each of the region's major sub-regions and nations. These discussions are premised on identification and discussion of many of the drivers of well-being discussed in this chapter but also include drivers that are unique to the discussions that are the focus of their chapter. The journey continues in the following Chap. 3 that examines the Economic Drivers.

References

Al-Azzawi, A. (2018). The Abbasids' house of wisdom in Baghdad. *Muslim Heritage: Discover the Muslim Golden Age of Muslim Civilization*. Retrieved September 19, 2018 from http://www.muslimheritage.com/article/abbasids-house-wisdom-baghdad.

Ali, A. & Al-Aswad, S. (2012). *Persian Gulf based SWFs & Financial Hubs in Bahrain, Dubai and Qatar: A Case of competitive branding*. Medford MA: Tufts University, Fletcher School. Retrieved October 23, 2018 from http://fletcher.tufts.edu/~/media/Fletcher/Microsites/swfi/pdfs/FINAL%20Asim-Shatha.pdf.

Bertman, S. (2005). *Handbook to life in ancient Mesopotamia*. New York and Oxford: Oxford University Press.

Central Intelligence Agency (CIA). (2018). *The world factbook*. Retrieved October 1, 2018 from https://www.cia.gov/library/publications/the-world-factbook/.

Charles River Editors, & Carabas, M. (2018). *Ra: The history and legacy of the ancient Egyptian God of the Sun*. Kindle Edition.

Clagett, M. (1999). *Ancient Egyptian science, a source book*—Vol. 3 *Ancient Egyptian mathematics*. Philadelphia American Philosophical Society.

Dodson, A. (2009). *Amarna Sunset: Nefertiti, Tutankhamun, Ay, Horemheb, and the Egyptian counter reformation*. Cairo: American University at Cairo.

Drews, R. (1995). *The end of the Bronze Age: Changes in warfare and the catastrophe Ca. 1200 B.C.* Princeton: Princeton University Press.

el-Aswad, el-S. (2019). Map of the North Africa and Middle East (MENA). Originally created by Amir el-Aswad as Figure 4.16 in Quality of Life and Policy Issues among the Middle East and North African Countries. Cham, Switzerland: Springer Nature International Publishers.

Encyclopedia Britannica. (2018). *Talion*. Retrieved October 24, 2018 from https://www.britannica.com/topic/talion.

Estes, R, J. (2019). The social progress of nations revisited, 1970–2020. *Social indicators research.* (in press).

Estes, R. J., & Tiliouine, H. (2016), Social development trends in the countries of the Fertile Crescent. In R. J. Estes, & H. Tiliouine. (Eds.), *Social progress in Islamic societies: Social, political, economic, and ideological challenges*. Chapter 9. Dordrecht NL: Springer International Publishers.

Estes, R. J., & Sirgy, M. J. (2014). Radical Islamic militancy and acts of terrorism: a quality-of-life analysis. *Social Indicators Research, 117*(2), 615–652.

Freedom House. (2018). *Freedom in the world*. New York: Freedom House.

Fund for Peace. (2018). *Failed states index, 2018*. Retrieved October 10, 2018 from http://fundforpeace.org/fsi/.

Gibbons, A. (2000). Jews and Arabs share recent ancestry. *Science.* Retrieved October 31, 2018 from https://www.sciencemag.org/news/2000/10/jews-and-arabs-share-recent-ancestry.

Gill, N. S. (2018, August 10). Who was Constantine the Great: His legacy including spreading Christianity through Roman Europe? *Thought Co.* Retrieved October 24, 2018 from https://www.thoughtco.com/constantine-the-great-112492.

Gordon, C. (1966). *The ancient near East* (3rd ed., Revised). New York: W. W. Norton and Company, Inc.

Gottlieb, A. (2017). *The dream of enlightenment: The rise of modern philosophy*. Meadville PA: Liveright.

Green, B. (2010). *Christianity in Ancient Rome: The first three centuries*. Bloomsbury: T & T Clark Publishers.

Gutas, D. (1998). *Greek thought, Arabic culture: The Graeco-Arabic translation movement in Baghdad and Early 'Abbāsid Society (2nd–4th/8th–10th Centuries)*, pp. 53–60. London: Psychology Press.

Guzman, G. (1985). Christian Europe and Mongol Asia: First Medieval intercultural contact between East and West. *Essays in Medieval Studies., 2,* 227–244.

Hammurabi & King, L. W. (2015). *The code of Hammurabi*. Various: CreateSpace Independent Publishing Platform.

Hancock, G. (2015). *Magicians of the gods*. New York & London: Thomas Dunne-Macmillan.

Hicks, E. & Hicks, J. (2007). *The teachings of Abraham book collection*. Carlsbad CA: Hay House.

Hillar, M. (2012). *From Logos to trinity. The evolution of religious beliefs from Pythagoras to Tertullian*. Cambridge: Cambridge University Press.

Imani, A. (2018). *The Muslim authoritarian mentality*. Retrieved October 8, 2018 from https://www.americanthinker.com/author/amil_imani/.

James, E. O. (1960). *The Ancient Gods: The history and diffusion of religion in the Ancient Near East and the Eastern Mediterranean*. New York: G.P. Putnam's Sons.

Kaplan, B. J. (2007). *Divided by faith: Religious conflict and the practice of toleration in early Modern Europe*. Cambridge MA: Belknap Press of Harvard University.

Kerr, R. (2011). *Christianity*. Retrieved October 1, 2018 from https://christianity.stackexchange.com/questions/3603/when-was-abraham-alive.

Keshavjee, M. M. (2016). Alternative Dispute Resolution (ADR) and its potential for helping Muslims reclaim the higher ethical values (Maqasid) underpinning the Sharia. In H. Tiliouine & R. J. Estes (Eds.), *Social progress in Islamic societies: Social, political, economic, and ideological challenges* (pp. 607–621). Dordrecht NL: Springer International Publishers.

Khan, A. O. (2018). List of prophets and their ages. Retrieved October 24, 2018 from http://educatebox.com/ages-of-prophets-list-of-prophets-and-their-ages/.

Krieger, B. (2016). *The Dead Sea and the Jordan River*. Bloomington: Indiana University Press.

Levine, A.-J. (2009). *The misunderstood Jew: The Church and the scandal of the Jewish Jesus*. New York: Harper One.

Lewis, B. (2003). *What went wrong: The clash between Islam and Modernity in the Middle East*. New York: Harper Perennial.

Lewis, C. S. (2017). Islam and the last battle. *PC New Speak Deconstruction*. Retrieved February 5, 2018 from https://pcnewspeak.blogspot.com/2017/05/cs-lewis-islam-and-last-battle.html.

Lewis, B., Holt, P., & Lambton, A. K. S. (1971). *The Cambridge history of Islam*. Cambridge: Cambridge University Press.

Liljas, A. E. M. (2015). Old age in ancient Egypt. *UCL: Researchers in the Museum*. Retrieved October 20, 2018 from https://blogs.ucl.ac.uk/researchers-in-museums/2015/03/02/old-age-in-ancient-egypt/.

Meier, J. P. (1991). *A Marginal Jew: Rethinking the historical Jesus*, v. 1–*The roots of the problem and the person*, Chapter 11, (pp. 373–433). New Haven: Yale University Press, Anchor Bible Reference Library.

National Consortium for the Study of Terrorism and Responses to Terrorism (START). (2018). *Database*. College Park: University of Maryland. Retrieved November 3, 2018 from https://www.start.umd.edu/.

Norland, R. (2017, November 8). An Iraqi town where religions coexist, in theory. *New York Times* A8. Retrieved from https://proxy.wm.edu/login?url; http://search.ebscohost.com/login.aspx?direct=true&AuthType=cookie,ip,url,shib&db=oih&AN=126097177&site=ehost-live&scope=site.

Organization of Islamic Cooperation (OIC). (2018). The collective voice of the Islamic world. Retrieved October 25, 2018 from https://www.oic-oci.org/home/?lan=en.

Plaut, W. G., & Bamberger, B. J. (1981). *The Torah—A modern commentary*. New York: Union of American Hebrew Congregations.

Raghavan, S. (2016). In post-Arab Spring Egypt, Muslim attacks on Christians are rising. *Washington Post*. Retrieved from https://www.washingtonpost.com/world/middle_east/in-post-arab-spring-egypt-muslim-attacks-on-christians-are-rising/2016/11/13/f50a18e2–84fc-11e6-b57d-dd49277af02f_story.html?noredirect=on&utm_term=.956c51f26c83 on February 28, 2019.

Religion of Peace. (2018). *What makes Islam so different: Forced conversion*. Retrieved October 5, 2018 from https://www.thereligionofpeace.com/pages/quran/forced-conversion.aspx.

Renima, A., Tiliouine, H., & Estes, R. J. (2016a). The Islamic golden age: A story of the triumph of the Islamic civilization. In Tiliouine, H., & Estes, R. J. (Eds.), *Social progress in Islamic societies: Social, political, economic, and ideological challenges.* Chapter 3. Dordrecht NL: Springer International Publishers.

Renima, A., Tiliouine, H., & Estes, R. J. (2016b). The changing map of the Islamic world: From the Abbasid Era to the Ottoman Empire of the 20th Century. In H. Tiliouine, & R. J. Estes (Eds.), *Social progress in Islamic societies: Social, political, economic, and ideological challenges.* Chapter 4. Dordrecht NL: Springer International Publishers.

River Valley Civilizations. (2017). *Tigris/Euphrates River Valley Civilization.* Retrieved November 2, 2018 from https://www.rivervalleycivilizations.com/tigris-euphrates.html.

Roudi, F. (2011). Youth population and employment in the Middle East and North Africa: Opportunity or challenge. *United Nations Expert Group Meeting on Adolescents, Youth and Development.* New York: UN Department of Economic and Social Affairs (DESA). Publication No. UN/POP/EGM-AYD/2011/06.

Schoch, R. (1992). Re-dating the Great Sphinx at Giza. *Circular Times Archives.* Retrieved October 1, 2018 from http://www.robertschoch.net/Redating%20the%20Great%20Sphinx%20of%20Giza.htm.

Shaikin, D., & Estes, R. J. (2018). Advancing development in Kazakhstan: The contribution of R&D. *Social Development Issues, 40*(2), 36–55. (20).

Sobhanbredin. (2018). Infinite present: Revelations from Islamic design in contemporary art. *Cambridge Community Television.* October 31. Retrieved November 3, 2018 from https://www.cctvcambridge.org/node/597124.

Stockholm International Peace Research Institute (SIPRI). (2018). *SIPRI yearbook 2018.* Stockholm: SIPRI. Available at https://www.sipri.org/yearbook/2018.

Tétreault, M. A., Okruhlik, G., & Kapiszewski, A. (Eds.). (2011). *Political change in the Arab Gulf States: Stuck in transition.* New York: Lynne Rienner Publishers.

Tiliouine, H., & Estes, R. J. (2016). *Social progress in Islamic societies: Social, political, economic, and ideological challenges.* Dordrecht NL: Springer International Publishers.

United Nations Development Programme (UNDP). (2018). *Human development report, 2018.* New York: UNDP.

Wikipedia. (2018a). *Semitic people.* Retrieved October 9, 2018 from https://en.wikipedia.org/wiki/Semitic_people.

Wikipedia. (2018b). *Forced coercion.* Retrieved November 8, 2018 from https://en.wikipedia.org/wiki/Forced_conversion.

Wilken, R. L. (2003). *The Christians as the Romans saw them* (2nd ed.). New Haven: Yale University of Press.

World Atlas. (2016). *Middle East Timeline.* Retrieved October 1, 2018 from https://www.worldatlas.com/webimage/countrys/asia/middleeast/metimeln.htm.

World Bank. (2018). *World development report, 2018: Learning to realize education's promise.* Washington: The World Bank Group. Retrieved October 15, 2018 from http://www.worldbank.org/en/publication/wdr2018.

Chapter 3
Joblessness, Political Unrest, and Jihadism Among the Region's Youth: Contemporary Challenges and Future Trends

Abstract The Middle East and North Africa region (MENA) has been one of the most economically dynamic in the world. The region's rate of economic expansion, due primarily to its rich oil and well-established human capital reserves, has been among the most robust of the world's 19 major subregions. And this historical pattern persists into the current period and is expected to continue to do so for at least the foreseeable future. This chapter explores the critical relationship that exists between the region's patterns of economic development and its broad-based social gains since the year 2000 to the present. Special attention is given to the relationship that exists between economic frustration, the region's rapidly increasing numbers of young people, the sense of relative deprivation experienced by these young people and, in some cases, their turning to violence, even terrorism, as an outlet for expressing their frustration and sense of aggrievement toward others they believe to be responsible for their poverty and, more fundamentally, sense of economic anomie. The chapter, however, is essentially positive in substance and projects a favorable future for most countries in the MENA region.

Keywords Economic drivers of jihadist terrorism · Youth unemployment · Economic development in MENA · Poverty in MENA countries · Economic anomie in MENA region

3.1 Introduction

Investment in education and economic prosperity is the best way to cure fanaticism and for establishing a just peace in the Middle East.

Ahmed Zewail[1]

Joblessness, political unrest and jihadism are closely intertwined with another, especially among the MENA's young people and recent university graduates who have not been able to secure suitable employment and incomes in their own societies (Fougère,

---

[1] https://www.brainyquote.com/quotes/ahmed_zewail_702624.

© Springer Nature Switzerland AG 2019
M. J. Sirgy et al., *Combatting Jihadist Terrorism through Nation-Building*, Human Well-Being Research and Policy Making, https://doi.org/10.1007/978-3-030-17868-0_3

Kramarz, & Pouget, 2009). The situation is especially serious in those of the region's nations for which their age dependency ratio exceeds 30% or even higher of a national population concentration, especially in countries in which the portion of children and youth are increasing at a rapid pace (United Nations, 2018). The contemporary situation is compounded within those countries that have high rates of aging populations in combination with limited numbers of economically active adults between the ages of 30 and 50 (50% or fewer) who can support their young, elderly, disabled and other financially dependent population groups (Tiliouine & Estes, 2016). Countries such as Afghanistan, Iran, Iraq, and Yemen simply are unable to provide for even the most basic material needs of their families or communities especially in that a disproportionate number of the region's societies are characterized by low or slow rates of economic expansion (International Monetary Fund, 2018; World Bank, 2018). High rates of inflation and military spending also impose severe restrictions on the social expenditures capacity of many of these nations, even for those with substantial levels of per capita income and steadily increasing rates of gross domestic product which use the bulk of their resources for infrastructure development.

Joblessness and high level of economic deprivation among the least advantaged in these societies are major drivers of jihadism in the region's diverse and multicultural population of approximately 411 million people, a very small portion of whom turn to violence to express their political, economic, or career frustration (Estes & Sirgy, 2015; Estes & Tiliouine, 2014; Filote, Potrafke, & Ursprung, 2016; Rahtz & Estes, 2019). Most of the violence-prone individuals are young but often function under the direction of older, usually highly educated, persons–some portion of which participated directly in violent activities when younger (Abu-Nimer & Hilal, 2016; Blaydes & Linzer, 2012). Not surprisingly, and as illustrated through the monograph, the leadership of many of these groups of young people are being led by university graduates who are unable to find acceptable forms of employment in countries where employment opportunities for recent university graduates are limited.

This chapter focuses on several underlying causes and contemporary expressions of the society-wide economic frustrations that exist within the MENA region that are closely associated with jihadism and to the rising levels of social and political conflict initiated by jihadists (Estes & Sirgy, 2018; Freytag et al. 2011; Richardson, 2013; World Bank, 2017):

(1) The overall economic "health" of the MENA region as reflected in rates of economic expansion, per capita growth and income levels, net wealth levels, employment and unemployment levels as well as poverty rates.[2]

(2) The relationships that exists between the region's demographic and economic trends with a focus on economic opportunity and other income security needs of the MENA rapidly increasing numbers of young people.

---

[2]Alphabetized List of MENA countries (Most commonly used): Algeria, Bahrain, Egypt, Iran (Islamic Republic of), Iraq, Israel, Jordan, Kuwait, Lebanon, Libya, Morocco, Oman, Qatar, Saudi Arabia, State of Palestine, Sudan, Syrian Arab Republic, Tunisia, Turkey, United Arab Emirates, Yemen.

(3) The relationship that exists between economic frustration in the region, espe-
     cially among its young people, and the growing sense of aggrievement, frustra-
     tion, and relative deprivation.
(4) The relationship between economic frustrations and violence including acts of
     local, national, regional, and international terrorism.
(5) The region's future economic outlook, again with special attention focused on
     its rapidly increasing population of young people, through to the years 2030
     and 2050.
(6) The presentation of some forward-looking suggestions that promote peaceful
     development via economic growth and a growing class of entrepreneurs—al-
     ways a strength among the region's diverse peoples.

All the content presented in this chapter builds on the region's contemporary
economic trends which has been well documented elsewhere by Estes & Tiliouine
(2014), Estes & Sirgy (2015, 2017, 2018, 2019a, 2019b), International Monetary
Fund (2018), International Social Security Association (2018), Tiliouine & Estes
(2016), World Bank (2018).

The substance of the chapter relates directly to the historical perspectives summarized by the author in Chap. 2 as well as the theoretical content of Chap. 1 and
the summary content of the monograph's concluding chapter (Estes & Sirgy, 2019a,
2019b). The major areas of emphasis of this chapter also overlap with those discussed
by Professor el-Sayed el-Aswad in his chapters that focus on the region's ancient
cultural history that have contributed so richly to the advancement of human civilization over several millennia (Estes & Sirgy, 2017; Tiliouine & Estes, 2016). More
particularly, the chapter focuses on (1) The MENA region's economic outlook to the
year 2025 and beyond (Estes, 2019c; World Bank, 2018); (2) short- and near-term
economic challenges in the MENA region (World Bank, 2013, 2018); (3) joblessness and economic frustration among the MENA region's young people, including
university graduates (ASDA'A Burson-Marsteller, 2018); and (4) looking back, but
moving forward: the ultimate economic challenges confronting the MENA region
(D'Cunha, 2017; Chaaban, 2010; Estes & Sirgy, 2019b). Though not representing
a complete list of the socioeconomic challenges that confront the MENA region,
nonetheless, the varied economic data discussed throughout the chapter present an
in-depth approach to promote a fuller explanation of that which exists in addition to
the many financial and economic issues that confront the Region's large number of
highly diverse group of nations (Estes & Sirgy, 2019a, 2019b; Sirgy, Joshanloo, &
Estes, 2019).

In commenting on the complexities associated with the type of socio-economic
research reported in this chapter, French economist Piketty (2015:130) observed,

> Social scientific research is and always will be tentative and imperfect. It does not claim to
> transform economics, sociology, and history into exact sciences. But by patiently searching
> for facts and patterns and calmly analyzing the economic, social, and political mechanisms
> that might explain them, it can inform democratic debate and focus attention on the right
> questions.

Note, too, that throughout the chapter, indeed throughout the monograph in its entirety, every effort has been made to limit the number of statistical tables and figures used to report complex numerical information and, instead, has sought to use words to report broad-based economic trends occurring in the MENA region. The intention of this decision was to make the major data patterns more accessible to the widest possible range of readers without requiring them to disaggregate complex statistical figures and tables that are reported by us elsewhere (Estes & Sirgy, 2015; Sirgy, Estes, & Rahtz, 2018). We have done so, however, without sacrificing the essential economic realities of the region and to cover region's long expanse of economic history with concentrations of great wealth but have placed emphasis on the years 2000 forward (Chaaban, 2010; Estes & Sirgy, 2015, 2019a, 2019b; Galasso, 2013; Hanushek, 2013; Hefner, 2014; International Monetary Fund, 2017a, 2017b, 2018).

This chapter contains just a few tables and figure. More detailed statistical data related to timely analytical patterns reported in this chapter have been summarized by the authors in other widely available academic publications (el-Aswad, 2016, 2019; Estes & Tiliouine, 2014; Estes & Sirgy, 2015; Sirgy et al. 2018; UN, 2016; UNCTAD, 2017; World Bank, 2017, 2018). Thus, readers have access to other descriptive and statistical data concerning the region's financial development over the recent past in two forms depending on their policy planning needs.

3.2 The MENA Region's Population (and Wealth Concentrations)

The MENA region is geographically large and both culturally and religiously diverse such that includes nation of North Africa and West Asia—commonly referred to as the "Middle East" (CIA, 2019). Afghanistan is not part of the MENA region but shares of the region's characteristics and, often, is included in more comprehensive discussions of the region. The region's size and cultural diversity has led to many significant accomplishments in the history of human civilization but also to conflict, especially given the concentration of wealth and large pockets of poverty, primarily in the region's countries with large concentrations of oil and fresh water (Hefner, 2014). The great wealth of this latter group of nations tends to be invested and reinvested in their own rather than foreign economies (Estes, 2019b; Estes & Sirgy, 2019a, 2019b). Many of the region's wealthiest countries, however, give generously to the support of their poorer neighbors especially in helping their citizens carry out at least one hajj to Mecca and to ensure the food they eat is halal and prepared according to Islamic principles. Of some interest, though, and rather ironically, levels of religiosity among all religious denominations living in the region's wealthier nations often tends to decline as level of economic growth rates and per capita income levels increase. These shifts are especially significant among those nations who are experiencing the most recent and rapid rates of economic expansion (Barber, 2013; IMF, 2018).

Some of the most important defining characteristics of the region's nations stem not only from differences that exist between them in terms of changing patterns of religiosity but also with respect to a wide range of cultural and economic characteristics (Estes, 2015, 2019a; Hanushek, 2013; IFAD, 2016; IMF, 2017b). Regarding language diversity, the OIC (2019:25) notes that there is not just one official language spoken in the region, albeit Arabic tends to unite these various linguistic groups. In all, there are five languages that are spoken predominately throughout the Middle East: Persian, Turkish, Arabic, Kurdish and Berber. After Arabic, Persian is the 2nd most frequently spoken language. English, however, is the predominate language used in commerce throughout much of the region and certainly the rest of the world.

3.2.1   The Six Most Populous Countries in the Middle East, 2016–2018

With a population of over 411 million people, it's easy to assume that there are extremely populated countries located in this region. Iran is by far the most populous, although Turkey is not far behind in numbers. The 3rd largest country, Iraq, has a population that is less than half of the observed numbers in Iran and Turkey, individually.

The MENA region's *six most populous countries* are identified in Table 3.1. As reflected on the four economic indicators reported for each of these countries their socio-political-economic characteristics are highly variable and contain data that are suggestive of the size of their geographic territories, their control over natural resources and even their degrees of political authoritarianism, levels of diversity-related social conflict, and extent of poverty and unemployment, especially for their violence-prone young people (Cruz, Quillin & Schellekens, 2015; Lozada, 2017; World Bank, 2013).

Although the actual numbers differ from those that characterized our base years of 2016–2018, the critical patterns reported in Table 3.1 for the four key economic measures have remained essentially the same, as have the joblessness patterns among the region's young people, a small percentage of which turn to violence as a way of expressing their sense of deprivation (CIA, 2019; World Population Review, 2018).

3.2.2   The MENA Region's Five Least Populous Countries in the Middle East, 2016–2018

The MENA region's five *least populous* countries of the MENA region are identified in Table 3.2. The same types of data reported in Table 3.1 for the region's most heavily populated nations are reported for its less populous nations as well. Though smaller than the countries identified in Table 3.1, the per capita Gross Domestic

Table 3.1 Selected economic characteristics of the MENA region's six most populous nations

Country	Population (Mil) 2019	Per capita GDP (PPP) 2017	National poverty rate 2017 (%)	Unemployment rate 2016 (%)
Egypt	100.5	$12,700	27.8	12.2
Iran	82.6	$20,100	18.7	11.8
Turkey	79.4	$27,000	21.9	10.9
Iraq	37.1	($2100)	14.0	16.0
Saudi Arabia	27.8	$54,500	NA	6.0
Yemen	26.7	$ 2500	54.0	27.1
Total	354.1			
Average	59.1	$19,117	27.3	14.0

Data Sources CIA (2019), IMF (2018), World Bank (2018), World Population Review (2018)

Table 3.2 Selected economic characteristics of the MENA region's five least populous nations

Country	Population (Mil) 2019	Per capita GDP (PPP) 2017	National poverty rate 2017	Unemployment rate 2016
Bahrain	1.4	$49,000	NA	3.6%
Qatar	2.2	$124,000	NA	8.9%
Kuwait	2.8	$65,800	NA	1.1%
Oman	3.3	$46,000	NA	NA
Lebanon	6.2	$19,600	28.6%	9.7%
Total	15.9			
Average	3.2	$69,088	NA	5.8

Data Sources CIA (2019), IMF (2018), World Bank (2018), World Population Review (2018)

Product (PPP)[3] is substantially higher on average, i.e., $69.1 thousand versus. $19.1 thousand for the region's more populous nations. The total population of the region's less populous nations are quite small in comparison with their nearby more populous countries, i.e., 15.9 million people versus a total of 354.1 million people in the region's most populous countries.

---

[3] *Purchasing power parity (PPP)* is an economic theory that compares different countries' currencies through a "basket of goods" approach. According to this concept, two currencies are in equilibrium or at par when a basket of goods (considering the exchange rate) is priced the same in both countries. Closely related to PPP is the law of one price, which is an economic theory that predicts that after accounting for differences in interest rates and exchange rates, the cost of something in country X should be the same as that in country Y in real terms (Investopedia, 2019).

3.2.3 *Egypt and Its Increasing Social and Economic Challenges*

The above characteristics are reflected in the region's diverse nations—both those that are small and those that are large. Egypt, for example, is the MENA region's most populous and for millennia culturally influential countries (CIA, 2019; Oakes & Gahli, 2018; Rutherford & Sowers, 2018), with a total population of more than 100,495,681 persons in February 2019 (Worldometers, 2019). The country's population growth rate ranges from 1.80 to 1.87% annually and approximately 39% of the country's population lives in urban communities—a number that is increasing rapidly such that approximately half of all Egyptians are expected to migrate to urban communities by as soon as 2030. This shifting population trend reflects the increased importance of manufacturing rather than agricultural jobs in supporting, and further increasing, the country's currently moderate level of economic expansion.

Viewed from another socioeconomic perspective, for two decades, many foreigners, despite the country's recent economic gains, believe that Egypt is a much too dangerous a country to visit, even as part of state-sponsored and supervised group tourism (Project Open Monograph, 1996). The country's recent turn to political authoritarianism and steadily increased levels of central government control over virtually all aspects of private life has added to Egypt's decendancy as a major center for tourism and for foreign direct investment (Egyptian News, 2019; Walsh, 2019). Recurrent violence directed at selected groups of Western countries also has reduced the countries attractiveness for many toward tourism, trade, and investment. The country's many ancient monuments and breathtaking museums has not been enough to offset the violence that permeates contemporary Egyptian society. Because of these factors, many people have lost jobs and the country's income from tourism and other sources have fall dramatically and likely will continue to do so until stability and peace are restored to the country. These critical drivers of economic development are essential to the future economic prospects of Egypt's very large population of young people who dependent on international investments to complete their education and, in time, attain well-paying job (Table 3.3).

The average size of Egyptian households is comparatively large by world standards at approximately 6–8 persons given that these households typically consist of three generations of family members (children, parents, and grandparents and, sometimes, others) with virtually all the household's economic responsibility assigned to its working age members aged between 17 and 60 years (for all but its disabled or otherwise limited family members). The size of Egyptian homes, however, are rather small given the highly expensive per capita and household costs associated with urban living in all the country's major cities.

Table 3.3 Population of Egypt (1990–2019)

Year	Population	Yearly % change (%)	Yearly change	Migrants (net)	Median age	Fertility rate	Urban pop (%)	Urban population	Country's share of world pop (%)	World population	Egypt global rank
2019	101,168,745	1.80	1,793,004	−55,000	24.8	3.33	38.7	39,172,736	1.31	7,714,576,923	14
2018	99,375,741	1.87	1,822,590	−55,000	24.8	3.33	38.7	38,491,949	1.30	7,632,819,325	14
2017	97,553,151	1.95	1,864,470	−55,000	24.8	3.33	38.8	37,826,341	1.29	7,550,262,101	14
2016	95,688,681	2.04	1,910,509	−55,000	24.8	3.33	38.9	37,175,090	1.28	7,466,964,280	14
2015	93,778,172	2.20	1,934,113	−55,005	24.7	3.38	39.0	36,537,834	1.27	7,383,008,820	14
2010	84,107,606	1.84	1,465,891	−56,715	23.9	2.98	39.9	33,587,708	1.21	6,958,169,159	15
2005	76,778,149	1.89	1,374,432	−14,893	22.6	3.15	40.2	30,883,800	1.17	6,542,159,383	15
2000	69,905,988	1.87	1,238,320	−42,180	21.2	3.41	40.5	28,304,150	1.14	6,145,006,989	15

Data Source Worldometers

3.3   The MENA Region's Population Pyramid

Population pyramids are constructed for graphically describing the distribution of a country's or region's population distribution by gender, age cohort, and the region-as-a-whole. Population pyramids also are used to capture irregularities in population distribution by age and gender but, primarily, those associated with age distributions.

Iran is the MENA region's second most populous country an estimated total of 83 million people. But not all Middle Eastern countries are so populous. However, all countries in the MENA region have populations that have surpass 1 million, and some of the least populous countries, such as Qatar, have an average annual growth rate that is up to 6 times as high, and even higher, than some of the MENA region's more populous areas.

3.3.1   Population Pyramid for Iran, 2014

The population pyramid shown below is for **Iran** in 2016 and was obtained from *Index Mundi* from the *World Fact Monograph* (Fig. 3.1). Box 3.1 reports Iran population distribution in 2016 by age, gender and percent of Iran's total population in 2016.[4]

Apart from its population size, Iran is one of the MENA region's most culturally homogenous, and politically influential countries that is also often the source of both regional and international social conflicts, including conflicts associated with the country becoming a nuclear state. The international conflicts, but especially those associated with the country's aggressive nuclear development program, have proven to be very significant and have resulted in the imposition of severe economic sanctions on the country by many Western nations, some of whom are nuclear powers in their own right, Western-imposed travel and economic sanctions on Iran, in turn, have added to the country's already high levels of joblessness and poverty and serves as the basis for violence-prone young and middle-aged persons to direct their frustrations toward both selected group in Iran and the MENA region as well as toward those Western states that have imposed the sanctions and, in doing so, brought about high levels of social misery, economic frustration, and heavy militarization of the country.

Iran's Age and Gender Distribution and their Economic Implications for the MENA Region: The age and gender distribution of the Iranian population in 2017 was: (1) *0–14 years*: 24.19% (male 10,154,424/female 9,690,512); (2) 15–24 years: 14.69% (male 6,174,435/female 5,878,475); (3) 25–54 years: 48.57% (male

---

[4]These entries provide the distribution of the population according to age. Information is included by sex and age group as follows: 0–14 years (children), 15–24 years (early working age), 25–54 years (prime working age), 55–64 years (mature working age), 65 years and over (elderly). The age structure of a population affects a nation's key socioeconomic issues. Countries with young populations (high percentage under age 15) need to invest more in schools, while countries with older populations (high percentage ages 65 and over) need to invest more in the health sector. The age structure can also be used to help predict potential political issues. For example, the rapid growth of a young adult population unable to find employment can lead to unrest.

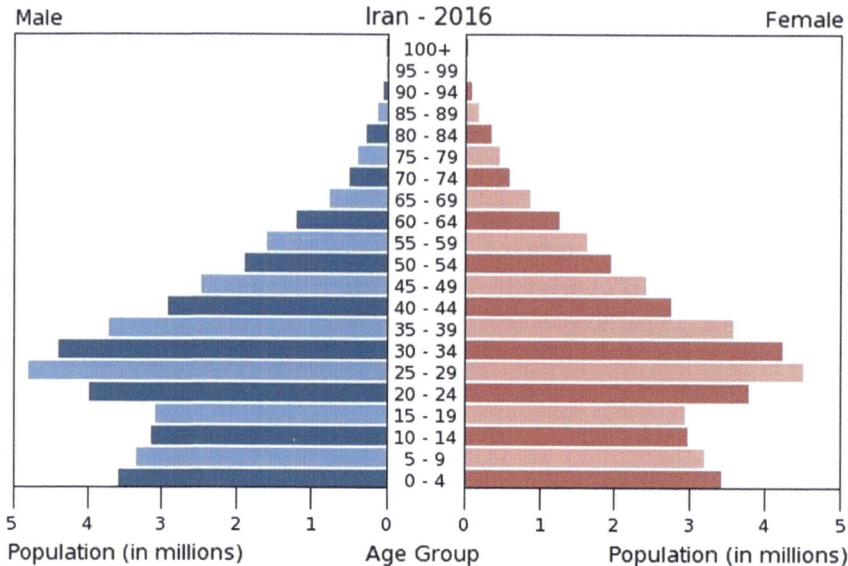

Fig. 3.1 Iran's population pyramid, 2016. *Source* Index Mundi: Iran. Retrieved February 15, 2019 from https://www.indexmundi.com/iran/age_structure.html. Copied from CIA World Factmonograph—This page was last updated on January 20, 2018. Available for free reproduction by the CIA (2018), Index Mundi (2019)

20,316,773/female 19,522,673); (4) 55–64 years: 7.22% (male 2,920,111/female 2,999,525); and, (5). 65 years and over: 5.32% (male 2,026,594/female 2,338,042). The country's total population 24 year of age and younger accounted for at least 39.0% of the country's total, the majority of whom were either too young to work or who were unable to find secure economic jobs for themselves (Fig. 3.1). The 15–24 age group is especially associated with Islamic Jihadism given the intense sense of deprivation, aggrievance, and sense of anomie that they experienced. These young people also were frequent initiators and, as they continued to age, targets of domestic and international violence as a way of expressing their acute sense of economic and social frustration (Bassiouni, 2016; Cruz, Quillin, & Schellekens, 2015; Estes & Sirgy, 2018; Lozada, 2017; World Bank, 2013).

Regional Economic Trends Associated with Iran's Demographic Pattern: Three demographic and related economic patterns that characterize the MENA region (and Iran using the above figure) are illustrated in the population pyramid presented for Iran in Fig. 3.1: (1) the regional and countries large numbers of young people below the age of 30 years; (2) an imbalance in the number of women to men as a result of male deaths associated with war, diversity-related and intraregional social conflicts (CIA, 2019; Hefner, 2014) and (3) Iran's comparatively small number of older and elderly population resulting, in the main, from limited family resources and highly constricted publicly financed social security and other related income security programs. All three of these patterns are troubling given the substantial oil reserves and other petroleum, agricultural, and mining products that are readily available from Iran from for trade in international markets. Given these resources, and the demands for them from international markets, one would have expected a very different set of social, political, and economic outcomes at both the local and national levels. But such has not been the case given the complex international and human capacity pressures that confront Iran daily with the result that social stagnation has come to characterize the nation over the past 25 years and longer (Barber, 2013).

3.3.2 Economic and Population-Related Social Deprivation in Iran and the Larger MENA Region

Iran is a heavily militarized society which, at the writing of this chapter, is celebrating its 40 years of authoritarian rule by the Shah and Shahin and their large network of officials, military officers, and its horrendous secret police, the Savak (Persian: ساواک, short for سازمان اطلاعات و امنیت کشور Sāzemān-e Ettelā'āt va Amniyat-e Keshvar, literally "Organization of National Intelligence and Security of the Nation") which committed unspeakable acts of terrorism against large segments of the economically disadvantaged population, including anomic students, clerics of other religious sects, and virtually anyone who spoke negatively of Shah or his regime.

This author tragically witnessed the deaths of hundreds of students and professors at the hands of the Savak and the Shah's military forces on the campus of the University of Teheran during the yearlong revolution that took place in the capital prior to the return of the Ayatollah Khomeini from Paris during the first months of 1979. These comparatively recent acts of brutality have remained in the hearts and minds of the Persians and, today, mirror themselves in similar events taking place in Syria, Iraq, and selected areas of other of the region's countries that border these nations.

Viewed from a Western perspective, much of the violence experience in Iran was supported through military training and munitions supplied by the United States during the decades of suffering experienced by the Persians at the hands of the Shah. The de-secularization of the country provided religious reunification for the country's almost totally Shi'a population (90%) and, from an economic perspective, the nationalization of the country's vast oil reserves and its other large markets made possible the steady accumulation of at least limited income and employment for larger numbers of Iranians, including Persian youth. Though this process is continuing to unfold many gains have been made by country which now has a per capital GDP of approximately $20,100 for those who are employed but, still, the country experiences extraordinarily high levels of unemployment (11.8% in 2017) and poverty (45–50%). These patterns also exist in other MENA countries that have experienced decades of social chaos—Afghanistan, Iraq, Syria, Yemen.

The following quote from an article written by Paige Frazier is illustrative of the sense of deep economic frustration experienced by Iran and selected other MENA countries that are confronting many of the same regional and international conflicts (Frazier, 2014, p. 2).

> A recent report titled *Measurement and Economic Analysis of Urban Poverty* showed that between 44.5 percent and 55.0 percent of Iran's urban population lives below the poverty line…The report did not include statistics for rural Iran…furthermore, 46 percent of Iranian women ages 15 to 24 are unemployed, and the unemployment rate for young adults is twice that of the general unemployment rate.

These profound economic problems continue to persist large because of the severe economic sanctions that have been placed on Iran its people by major Western powers with the United States providing the leadership for these sanctions. The sanctions have been imposed because of violence and acts of state-sponsored terrorism that is attributed to Iran and other countries allied with Iran. Iran's insistence in developing its own nuclear resources has added to the tensions experienced by Western nations given the fear that such developments will be targeted by Iran against European and North American nations who are regarded as the most serious enemies of the country.

The Iranian economic and political reality is not unique to the MENA region. Many of the same dynamics are operating between Western nations and those Syria, Iraq, and Afghanistan—all three of which are struggling with decades of especially lethal civil wars and diversity-related social conflict.

3.4 The MENA Region's Economic Outlook to 2050

Overall, and despite the recurrent economic problems experienced by the countries in conflict, the MENA region is one of the world's wealthiest and most advantaged in terms of national resources that are in great demand. There is currently no reason for believing that this general pattern will change appreciably especially as the region human resource capacities continue to increase and become more influential across the world. Certainly, these patterns will persist until at least 2050 as an increasing number of economically advanced nations in all regions of the world continue to invest in the region's development (International Monetary Fund, 2017a, 2017b). General patterns reported in 2017 are likely to be retained over the near time. For example,

- Rates of GDP are likely to remain the same over the foreseeable near-term thus, adding, to the region's wealth of nations.
- Income levels are likely to continue to increase over at least the near-term, albeit are expected to increase at the same rate as have taken place since at least 2015.
- The national rates of economic growth will remain the same for at least the near term.
- Rates of inflation, as in the rest of the economically advanced word, is expected to remain comparatively low at well below 5% between 2015 and 2020.

- Per capita income levels are expected to remain stable for at least the next decade though more rapid rates of economic growth would substantially decrease the levels of jihadism associated with this pattern of economic growth.
- These patterns are expected to differ appreciably from one group of nations in the region to another but, nonetheless, the region's economic pattern of expected continued group should continue to occur as anticipated.

3.5   Current Economic Trends in the MENA Region

The economics of the MENA region are quite complex given the region's scarce natural resources and its concentration of primarily oil and, in recent years, financial services within selected countries of the region. As elsewhere in the world, the region's economic consists of six level of economic well-being: (a) Individuals, families, and extended kinship systems; (b) local neighborhoods and communities; (c) states and provinces; (d) nations; (e) major world geopolitical regions; and, (f) the world-as-a-whole. These six levels of economic well-being add to both the richness of the region's economies and provide the reader with a fuller understanding of the economic drivers that form the region's comprehensive wealth and poverty development.

The region's six levels of economic development are significantly influenced by diversity-related social conflicts, civil wars, intraregional wars and other conflicts that several constrain the region's pace of economic expansion. This situation is especially serious within those nations that have been classified internationally as either "failed" or "failing states" (Ingersoll & Jones, 2013). International foreign development assistance to the region's nations engaged in recurrent internal and intraregional conflicts and, in turn, have added to the unique challenges confronted by the nations of the MENA region as it seeks to modernize its often ancient, in some cases authoritarian social, political and economic systems (CIA, 2019; OIC, 2018). The region also struggles with issues of political and press freedom and many nations outside of the region is its propensity for violence, civil wars, and international conflicts.

As of the writing of this chapter, the economies of many of the region's most competitive economies has experienced very low levels of economic growth combined with high levels of jobless and inflation (el-Aswad, 2019). According to an estimate by *FocusEconomics*, the MENA economy expanded by an aggregate 1.8% annually in Q3 (Torné, 2019). These levels were well below both Q2's 2.1% expansion and the 2.0% rise projected for January 2019. That said, Iran represented the lion share of the slowdown in Q3 as the country was negatively affected by the reintroduction of economic sanctions by the United States. However, and according to *FocusEconomics* in February 2019,

> …economic dynamics among the oil-exporting countries, excluding Iran, gained steam in Q3 on the back of stronger oil production and rising oil prices. Nevertheless, this trend likely came to an end in Q4 due to the sharp drop in oil prices observed since mid-October and

reduced oil production in December ahead of the oil cap deal, which came into effect in January 2019. Economic growth among oil-importing nations seems to have decelerated slightly in Q3…hat said, solid domestic demand, a healthy influx of tourists and robust agricultural production allowed growth to remain robust overall. (Torné, 2019, p. 2)

3.6 A Region in Economic Crisis

Unfortunately, and despite many positive economic gains, economic growth for the Middle East and North Africa as a whole is continuing to quickly deteriorate despite the reality that the international oil led by OPEC appears to be stable and like will remain so through the greater part of 2019. While the OPEC arrangement has the potential to increase oil prices, it will likely reduce both crude oil volumes among oil-exporting nations and the income from what that do receive from the sale of this critical regional resource. However, higher oil prices will erode households' purchasing power and reducing fiscal space. Global financial conditions are gradually tightening with major central banks starting to control monetary stimulus, which threatens to heighten volatility in the region's financial markets. The U.S. Federal Reserve's conservative approach at its January 2019 meeting, however, should usher in a period of calm, at least until the end of its H1 period (Board of Governors of the Federal Reserve System, 2019).

Political unrest remains elevated with protests spreading across the region. Long-standing sectarian conflicts, with Yemen as the paradigm; widespread poverty; and stagnating progress in social and economic reforms seem to be igniting the region. Recurrent civil unrest in Syria, Iraq, and, to lesser extent, Iran also are contributing to the region's major economic, social, and political challenges and are not likely to be resolved in the near term—especially given the proliferation of Jihadist forces functioning in and near these countries. Certainly, opportunities for economic expansion in these heavily populated Shia nations is not expected to change at any time in the foreseeable future given the multiple drivers that have sustained these conflicts even as Iran is currently celebrating the 40th anniversary of the downfall of the Shah and the emergence of a new *Islamic Republic of Iran* in which religion and religious leaders are central to its governance (Ali, 2016). Despite the country's vast oil reserves, it remains poor with weak infrastructure in combination with high levels of poverty and unemployment.

Panelists associated with the highly influential *FocusEconomics Consensus Forecast* expect the region to expand 1.9% in 2019, which is down 0.2 percentage points from last month's estimate, and 2.8% in 2020. The 2019 growth projections for Algeria, Bahrain, Iraq, Jordan, Kuwait, Lebanon, Morocco, Oman, Qatar, Saudi Arabia, Tunisia, the UAE and Yemen were revised downwards this month. In contrast, the forecast for Egypt was revised up, while estimates for Iran and Israel saw their 2019 estimates unchanged. Egypt is expected to be the region's top performer in 2019, followed by Iraq. Iran will also contract further in fiscal year 2019 as U.S. sanctions continue to limit the country's ability to engage in international trade (Torné, 2019).

   While the economy of Saudi Arabia appears to have ended 2018 on a solid footing, prospects for 2019 and 2020 are quickly deteriorating. By contrast, the Israeli economy accelerated strongly in the third quarter from limited growth rate recorded in the second quarter.

   Economic growth in Egypt grew at a strong but unchanged pace in the second quarter of fiscal year 2019—which covered October to December 2018—following a small slowdown in the first quarter. Although comprehensive data is outstanding, this came on the heels of increased investment (Sehgal, 2017). Moreover, the government expects unemployment to have fallen in the same period, which, combined with higher public-sector pay, likely supported private consumption growth.

   Economic growth across the entire MENA region should be solid and sustainable over the near term despite the variations that have occurred in regional countries that have experienced years, indeed decades, of deterioration associated with civil and intraregional work and, in recent years, international conflicts (United Nations, 2017a, 2017b; UNDESA, 2017). Inflation levels in these countries are likely to fall and to continue to descend over several years of economic development (Todaro & Smith, 2012). The projection is that inflation for the region will average 7.2% in 2019, down 0.1 percentage points from each month throughout 2018. In 2020, regional inflation is expected to decline to 5.6%.

3.6.1   *Joblessness, Entrepreneurs, and Economic Frustration Among the MENA Region's Young People, Including University Graduates*

The region's young people are especially vulnerable to high rates of chronic joblessness much of last for many years. This forces most young people to live with their families of origin, reduce the likelihood of finding suitable marriage partners, and live at subsistence levels of well-being. Many of these young people engage in petty theft and more serious acts of thefts in order to provide for not only their basic needs but more advanced electronic and other expensive goods and services as well, including travel to other countries in the region. See the case in Egypt (Box 3.1).

Box 3.1: Economic Issues in Egypt: Grand Plans Versus Grass Roots

High unemployment among youth in Egypt is a good example of the need to invest in long term solutions to economic issues. Ghafar (2016) notes that if the government does not deal with this major social and economic issue, it will face a potentially very unpleasant future. It seems, however, that high profile, high cost, grandiose infrastructure projects are at the center of the Egyptian economic plan. A quick snapshot shows the Egyptian currency under stress, and grand plan infrastructure projects failing to deliver on promises of systemic positive economic impact. A proposed new capital outside of Cairo, is foundering, and the widening of the Suez Canal for $8 Billion, touted as a $100 Billon revenue generator after one year of operation, has yet to come near such projections as shipping conglomerates still use the longer, but much cheaper transit routes to markets around the world. There is no easy answer to causes of the youth unemployment problem in Egypt. Two significant contributors, however, are quite clear. A higher education system that graduates thousands, but an Egyptian economy that cannot absorb the graduates into the graduate's field of study. That be a mismatch between education and industry skill set demands among other things. The second of these factors is basic demography. There is a large and growing youth population bulge in Egypt. As an outcome of this you again have a labor pool that cannot find desired types of jobs, or even any job. Between 1998 and 2006 alone, the age cohort of 15–29 increased from 17.4 million to 22.2 million. That number is not slowing down, it is increasing. One of the drivers of Islamist success in recruitment is economics based. The government must further invest in an education system that matches industry demands. It is the type of long-term national investment that reaches down to the local needs of its people for better opportunities in employment and quality of life.

Adapted from: Ghafar (2016).

Derek Thompson, a staff writer who concentrates on economic affairs for *The Atlantic Magazine,* suggests that a variety of fundamental macro and microeconomic factors influence one's perception of happiness, including those populations endemic to the MENA region: (1) richer countries are happier countries; (2) richer people are happier people; (3) but money has diminishing returns—like just about everything else; (4) income inequality reduces well-being, and higher public spending increases well-being; (5) unemployment makes you miserable; (6) inflation makes you unhappy, too; (7) working more hours makes you happier … until it doesn't; (8) commuters are less happy; (9) self-employed people are happier; and, (10) debt sucks (Thompson, 2012).

Thompson's somewhat humorous written article captures of essence of many much longer treatises, including as the relationship that exists between economic and younger working age persons in the MENA region. His summary, however, does not capture the region's history of violence in response to long-term economic insecurity, especially the chronic lack of paid employment for the region's youth including many of its rapidly increasing number of university graduates. Nor do his comments reflect the forced choice made by many of the region's young people to enter military service as an approach for dealing with their long-term under- and unemployment. For many young people this choice does open career opportunities for many young people that otherwise would not be available, especially if they learn new skills. Military service also often confers on enrollee's special status within both their families and communities as well, especially if there exists a family history of national military service to the country. Though only a comparatively small amount, past and current military service does provide many of the region's young people with at least modest levels of economic support over extended time periods, including to those who have experienced serious injuries during service or, in extreme situations, to their families should the service member be killed during military service to the nation.

Women are especially included in the group of employment seeking applicants but, as in the past, most of their employment opportunities remain restricted to gender-associated positions as teachers, nurses, in light industry but, increasing in comparable positions in the military as well. Illiterate persons and persons with low skill sets, when, such jobs exist, engage in heavy manufacturing, mining and other extraction work, as janitors and building cleaners and the like. A very large share of these persons enters the military as well and experience extraordinarily high mortality rates which also deprives their countries of much valued human resources.

Other young people, including disproportionate numbers of young women, do, of course, also delay their entry in the labor force through enrollment in institutions of higher learning, most of which are available at very low costs to qualified students (ASDA'A Burson-Marsteller, 2018).

Still other young people, including women, have turned to their own skills to create jobs and businesses from which reliable levels of income could be made, often at levels comparable to higher than that earned by others working in the region's extensive network of oil-exporting (West Asia) and powerful financial centers located in the Gulf States. Many of these businesses are established on ones that already had been created by members of their extended kinship networks, especially at the retail level, but others were established through partnerships with other young people with the help of financially-oriented international development assistance organizations, via loans provided by specialized governmental and business enterprises and, in the case of large businesses, through fund made available via *Foreign Direct Investment* (FDI) entities (International Monetary Fund, 2017a, 2017b; Sehgal, 2017).[5]

As is the case in most societies, many of these upstart businesses, whether started by younger or older entrepreneurs, fail in their early years but others go on to succeed in achieving high levels of success that eventually create job opportunities for many young people. These far-reaching economic trends are impressive and reflect favorably on the willingness of the region's young people to take on and overcome substantial investment risks (of time, talent, and both fiscal and human capital). Manufacturing, electronic, real estate, and the provision of consulting and other service enterprises proved to be especially successful in the region's countries which high

---

[5]Global inflows of foreign direct investment (FDI) fell by 18% in 2012 to $1.35 trillion, as the world economy slowed and political uncertainty in some big economies made investors cautious. The European Union alone accounted for two-thirds of this decline. Inflows to developed countries fell by a third to $561 billion, the lowest for almost a decade. Developing countries received 52% of global inflows, overtaking rich countries for the first time. Although the overall amount of investment to developing economies fell slightly, some regions performed strongly. South America's inward FDI rose by 12%, and Africa's by 5%. And inflows to the world's poorest countries hit a record high (Economist, 2017).

levels of previously displaced economic entrepreneurs who were able to establish at least small and medium sized businesses. Young entrepreneurs interested in establishing larger business enterprises typically migrate to nearby, more economically advanced, countries to establish their businesses or to enter into partnerships with already established entrepreneurs located in the migrant-receiving country(ries). This well-established pattern of economic entrepreneurism among migrating Arabs has persisted for centuries and continues to strength the economic human capacity of many of the region's most talented business leaders (Estes, 2019a, 2019b).

3.6.2 Other Major Economic Challenges Confronting the MENA Region

The economic trends confronting the MENA region are complex, demanding, and require substantial national and regional effort to resolve: (1) slow to moderate levels of economic expansions; (2) comparatively high to moderate level of chronic unemployment that affects large segments of the total population of a nation and the larger region; (3) restricted level of intraregional and international trade; (4) comparatively highly levels of inflation that last over a long time period; (5) reduced patterns of international trade for the scarce goods that already are produced by the MENA region; (6) continuing weak, certainly uneven, social security and other programs of income security for especially vulnerable population groups; and, (7) high levels of public expenditures for defense and military purposes which render even more complex solutions to the multiple levels of social challenges identified in the above items (el-Aswad, 2019). The absence of dependable sources of financial resources to resolve all seven of these recurrent national and regional challenges have rendered resolution of all seven-challenge confronting the MENA regions among the most difficult in the world.

   No evidence exists for believing that these highly complex demands on the growth trends of the region's nations can be resolved without substantial international development assistance, including that created through the creation of international businesses in the region including those established through foreign direct assistance. These solutions have worked well in other groups of nations (World Bank, 2018) and almost certainly will function to reduce the high levels of chronic unemployment, especially among young people, that is a major feature of the region's overall pattern of socioeconomic development (ASDA'A Burson-Marsteller, 2018; D'Cunha, 2017: May 11). Terrorism and international violence play no role in ensuring the success of these mostly innovative and businesses that engage in both national and international transactions for which a high level of cooperation is required (Czinkota, Knight, Liesch, & Steen, 2010).

3.7 Economic Frustration, Violence, and Terrorism

As will be discussed throughout this monograph a close relationship exists between low income and a psychological sense of relative deprivation. This sense of relative deprivation can be very profound and, not infrequently, contributes to expression of anti-social behavior that is expressed toward others, sometimes through violence. Often, these violent actions are expressed toward family members, often toward spouses and children, but, in time, these feelings of deprivation are expressed to others in the community and, in the most egregious situations, toward members of already historically disadvantaged groups, including toward religious minorities. This form of economic deprivation also can, and often is, directed through gang behavior which targets similar population groups in other nearby nations and, in extreme situations, toward people and institutions (political and financial) located in more economically advanced nations that are believed to be the underlying source of the economic maladies that confront populations in selected less economically developed MENA region (Bassiouni, 2016; Kinzer, 2003; Rahtz & Estes, 2019).

3.8 Looking Back, but Moving Forward: The Ultimate Economic Challenges Confronting the MENA Region

The MENA region is a highly dynamic region and among one of the most dynamic of the world's 19 major subregions worldwide (Estes, 2019b, 2019c). The region's general economic health is very favorable and current trends suggest that rates of economic growth, in combination with increasing diversity of products using the region's limited natural resource base of agricultural products as well as extraction services including the production of oil and related petroleum products. The MENA region also is a major exporter of contract labor of at semi-skilled workers to neighboring countries for mostly building and oil extraction work and the remittances sent by these workers to their families at home add substantially to the region's economic growth for both worker sending and receiving counties (Pettinger, 2013; World Bank, 2014, 2016). Unfortunately, the region also has a high rate of outmigration to a broad range of countries in Europe and North America, but this trend is resulting in substantial losses to the MENA send countries in well-educated and often experienced professional young people from countries that desperately require such skills to promote their own national (and regional) development associated with the same potentially high-priced skills. Though these migratory trends are helping to promote the region's economies the real need is for these skilled human capital resources to contribute to the economies of their own nations (Pettinger, 2013; Piketty, 2013). As suggested by French economist Thomas Piketty in his monograph *Capital in the 21st Century*,

> Over a long period of time, the main force in favor of greater equality has been the diffusion of knowledge and skills. (p. 150)

Further, other countries, especially those that already are economically develop-ment, need to participate more actively in the economic development of the MENA region's highly diverse nations. Technical and financial assistance toward these coun-tries are especially needed this point in their economic history as is the need for Foreign Direct Investment (FDI) (Editors, 2013; Sehgal, 2017; Shah, 2014; USAID, 2007), bi- and multi-lateral agreements between the region's poorer nations and those that are more economically advantaged, including more distant countries in the world's more economically advantaged regions that traditionally have been major contributors to the development of these countries[6] (Kilmister, 2016; OECD, 2015, 2016a, 2016b; Shah, 2014).

3.9 Discussion

The Middle East and North Africa region (MENA) has been one of the most econom-ically dynamic in the world. The region's rate of economic expansion, due primarily to its rich oil reserves and well-established human capital reserves, have been among the most robust of the world's 19 major subregions. And this historical pattern per-sists into the modern era and is expected to continue to fuel the region's positive economic development well into the future (Estes, 2019b; Todara & Smith, 2012).

But the MENA region's approximately 411 million people, substantially larger if one includes Afghanistan (as other often do because of its many shared characteristics with the group of usually identified MENA states), are characterized by high levels of diversity-related and social conflict, including intraregional conflicts and outright wars.

These conflicts are very troubling for the region and, in the main, serve as a dis-couragement for nations outside of the region to assist them, including in the form of technical and financial assistance, cultural and scholarly exchanges, and other forms of interaction which foster a sense of cooperation and peace in contributing to infrastructure development of many countries and other regions around the world. These conflicts unfortunately are closely associated with the region's rapidly increas-ing number of young people, including university graduates who cannot find secure employment for themselves, that undermine both the nature and pace of economic development between and within the region's highly diverse nations (Landis, 2015). These conflicts are extremely serious and for more than two decades has resulted in acts of internal and international violence, including acts of terrorism directed at

---

[6]In recognition of the special importance of the role which can be fulfilled only by official develop-ment assistance, a major part of financial resource transfers to the developing countries should be provided in the form of official development assistance (Shah, 2014). Each economically advanced country will progressively increase its official development assistance to the developing countries and will exert its best efforts to reach a minimum of 0.7% of its gross national product at market prices by the middle of the decade (Organization for Economic Cooperation and Development, 2018).

Western capital cities and economic centers have are believed to be the source of economic frustration and stagnation in some area of the MENA region.

Bassiouni, 2016; el-Aswad, 2016, 2019; Estes & Sirgy, 2015, 2019a, 2019b; Ferrero, 2005; Keshavjee, 2016; Krieger & Meierrieks, 2011; Kurrild-Klitgaard et al., 2006; Law, 2015; Rahtz & Estes, 2019 among many other scholars, have devoted considerable attention to this issue and have proposed a wide range of solutions consistent with Islamic values that are intended to reduce the incidence of terrorist behavior toward intraregional and international conflict. Major economic sanctions have been applied to selected subgroups of MENA nations but the results, to date, has not proven effective. The new, often innovative, approaches to economic development through peace promotion have not yet taken hold with the results that rates of economic growth, employment and international trade has been reduced substantially including support for these economies through traditional sources of international development assistance. The net result of all these trends is one of comparative economic stagnation except for the continuing moderate to high levels of economic expansion continuing to be experienced by the region's major oil exporting and still emerging regional banking countries located primarily in the natural resource poor but human capital rich Gulf States.

Many positive solutions to the region' economic conundrum have been offered and still more and being developed by the region's steadily younger political leaders. These include resolving some of the chronic political problems that have confronted the region's nation, advanced the economic capacity of selected subpopulations of the long ignored women, developing the beginning of a publicly funded, certainly sponsored, social welfare networks to address the economic needs of the region's most income insecure populations, as well as building better transportation, communications, housing and other elements of critical infrastructure that will unite an increasing larger share of the region's rapidly increasing population, especially its disproportionate numbers of child and youth who will eventually move into the region's major leadership positions (ASDA'A Burson-Marsteller, 2018; D'Cunha, 2017). The attainment of these goals is essential to reducing the region's level of social conflict and improving its happiness scores as measure by international metrics (Clark & Senik, 2017; Helliwell, Layard & Sachs, 2017; Thompson, 2012). The attainment of both objectives will significantly advance the MENA region's pattern of economic expansion as well. The MENA region, in combination with other comparatively low-income world, in the end, is expected to contribute to rates of global economic expansion which is expected to total at least 60% of all world economic growth (OECD, 2017; Stiglitz, 2015). The MENA region, given its vast oil reserves, is likely to account for a disproportionately high percentage of world economic growth that can be attributed to sustained economic growth of all low-income and socially least developing countries (Vanham, 2015). This is a very optimistic view of the region's near-term economic development indeed. We shall watch and contribute our own efforts to help bring this about.

References

Abu-Nimer, M., & Hilal, M. (2016). Combatting global stereotypes of Islam and Muslims: strategies and interventions for mutual understanding. In H. Tiliouine & R. J. Estes (Eds.), *The state of social progress of Islamic societies: Social, political, economic and ideological challenges*. Dordrecht NL: Springer.

Ali, L. (2016). *British diplomacy and the Iranian revolution, 1978–1981*. London: Palgrave Macmillan.

ASDA'A Burson-Marsteller. (2018). *Ten years of Arab youth survey: A decade of hopes and fears*. Dubai: Dubai Media City. Retrieved February 9, 2019 from http://www.arabyouthsurvey.com/.

Barber, N. (2013). Country religiosity declines as material security increases. *Cross-Cultural Research, 47*(1), 42–50.

Bassiouni, M. C. (2016). Islam and contemporary violence: A historic turning point. In H. Tiliouine & R. J. Estes (Eds.), *Social progress in Islamic societies: Social, political, economic, and ideological challenges*. Dordrecht NL: Springer International Publishers.

Blaydes, L., & Linzer, D. A. (2012). Elite competition, religiosity, and anti-Americanism in the Islamic World. *The American Political Science Review, 106*(2), 225–243.

Board of Governors of the Federal Reserve System. (2019). *Factors affecting reserve balances—H.4.1*. Washington: Board of Governors of the Federal Reserve System. Retrieved February 11, 2019 from https://www.federalreserve.gov/releases/h41/.

Central Intelligence Agency (CIA). (2019). *World factmonograph, 2019*. Retrieved February 9, 2019 from https://www.cia.gov/library/publications/the-world-factmonograph/.

Chaaban, J. (2010). *Job creation in the Arab economies: Navigating through difficult waters*. United Nations: Regional Bureau for Arab States, Research Paper #3. Retrieved February 4, 2019 from http://arab-hdr.org/publications/other/ahdrps/paper03-en.pdf.

Clark, A., & Senik, C. (2017). *Happiness and economic growth: Lessons from developing countries*. Oxford: Oxford University Press.

Cruz, M., Quillin, B., & Schellekens, P. (2015). *The three major challenges to ending extreme poverty*. Washington, DC: World Bank.

Czinkota, M. R., Knight, G., Liesch, P. W., & Steen, J. (2010). Terrorism and international business: A research agenda. *Journal of International Business Studies, 41*, 826–843.

D'Cunha, S. D. (2017, May 11). Plagued by a 30% unemployment rate, Arabian youth turn to startups for a lifeline. *Forbes*. Retrieved February 9, 2019 from https://www.forbes.com/sites/suparnadutt/2017/05/11/can-startups-drive-new-job-growth-in-the-mena-region-where-youth-unemployment-rate-is-30/#53dc08e534f4.

Editors. (2013, June 29). Foreign direct investment by major world region, 2007–2012. *The Economist*. Retrieved January 13, 2017, from http://www.economist.com/news/economic-and-financial-indicators/21580200-foreign-direct-investment.

Egyptian News. (2019). Breaking local news. *Egyptian Breaking News*, Retrieved February 15, 2019 from www.getlocalnewsnow.co/News/Egypt.

el-Aswad, el-S. (2016). Political challenges confronting the Islamic world. In H. Tiliouine & R. J. Estes (Eds.), *The state of social progress of Islamic societies: Social, economic, political, and ideological Challenges* (pp. 361–377). AG Switzerland: Springer International Publishing.

el-Aswad, el-S. (2019). *The quality of life and policy issues among the Middle East and North African Countries*. New York: Springer Nature Switzerland AG.

Estes, R. J. (2015). Development trends among the world's socially least developed countries: Reasons for cautious optimism. In B. Spooner (Ed.), *Globalization: The crucial phase*. Philadelphia: University of Pennsylvania Press.

Estes, R. J. (2019a). Disparities and wealth. In G. Brule & C. Suter (Eds.), *Wealth and subjective well-being*. Dordrecht NL: Springer International Publishers.

Estes, R. J. (2019b). The social progress of nations revisited. *Social Indicators Research*, 34 pages. https://doi.org/10.1007/s11205-018-02058-9.

Estes, R. J. (2019c). *The social progress of nations revisited: Fifty years of promise and progress.* Cham, Switzerland: Springer Nature International Publishers. in press.

Estes, R. J., & Sirgy, M. J. (2015). Radical Islamic militancy and acts of terrorism: a quality-of-life analysis. *Social Indicators Research, 117*(2), 615–652.

Estes, R. J., & Sirgy, M. J. (Eds.). (2017). *The pursuit of well-being: The untold global history.* Dordrecht NL & Berlin: Springer International Publishers.

Estes, R. J., & Sirgy, M. J. (2018). *Advances in well-being: Toward a better world for all.* London: Rowman and Littlefield.

Estes, R. J., Sirgy, M. J. (2019a). Global advances in quality of life and well-being: Past, present, and future. *Social Indicators Research, 141*(3), 1137–1164.

Estes, R. J., & Sirgy, M. J. (2019b). Advances in well-being in the MENA region: Accentuating the positive. In L. Lambert & N. Pasha-Zaidi (Eds.), *Advances in well-being in the Middle East and North Africa (MENA) region: Historical background and contemporary challenges.* Dordrecht: Springer International Publishers.

Estes, R. J., & Tiliouine, H. (2014). Islamic development trends: From collective wishes to concerted actions. *Social Indicators Research, 116*(1), 67–114.

Ferrero, M. (2005). Radicalization as a reaction to failure: An economic model of Islamic extremism. *Public Choice, 122*(1/2), 199–220.

Filote, A., Potrafke, N., & Ursprung, H. (2016). Suicide attacks and religious cleavages. *Public Choice, 166*(1/2), 3–28.

Fougère, D., Kramarz, F., & Pouget, J. (2009). Youth unemployment and crime in France. *Journal of the European Economic Association, 7*(5), 909–938.

Frazier, P. (2014). Poverty in Iran on the rise. *Borgen Magazine.* Retrieved February 13, 2019 from https://www.borgenmagazine.com/poverty-iran-rise/.

Freytag, A., Kruger, J. J., Meierrieks, D., & Schneider, F. (2011). The origins of terrorism: Cross-country estimates of socio-economic determinants of terrorism. *European Journal of Political Economy, 27,* S5–S16.

Galasso, V. N. (2013). *The drivers of economic inequality: A primer.* Washington, DC: Oxfam USA. Retrieved April 3, 2017, from https://www.oxfamamerica.org/static/media/files/oxfam-drivers-of-economic-inequality.pdf.

Ghafar, A. A. (2016). *Youth unemployment in Egypt: A ticking time bomb.* Brookings Institution. Retrieved from https://www.brookings.edu/blog/markaz/2016/07/29/youth-unemployment-in-egypt-a-ticking-time-bomb/# on February 28, 2019.

Hanushek, E. A. (2013). *Economic growth in developing countries: The role of human capital.* Palo Alto: Hoover Institution.

Hefner, R. (2014). Islam and plurality, old and new. *Society, 51*(6), 636–644.

Helliwell, J., Layard, R., & Sachs, J. (2017). *World happiness report, 2017.* New York: Sustainable Development Solutions Network.

Index Mundi. (2019). *Population pyramid for Iran, 2012 by gender and age group.* Retrieved February 16, 2019 from https://www.indexmundi.com/iran/age_structure.html.

Ingersoll, G., & Jones, B. (2013). The 25 most failed states on earth. *Business Insider,* July 11. Retrieved February 10, 2019 from https://www.businessinsider.com/the-25-most-failed-states-on-earth-2013-6.

International Fund for Agricultural Development (IFAD). (2016). *Reaching the Rural Poor.* Rome: IFAD. Retrieved January 23, 2017 from https://www.ifad.org/documents/10180/dc9da3d9-b603-4a9a-ba67-e248b39cb34f.

International Monetary Fund (IMF). (2017a). *Comparative world economic outlook, 2018.* Retrieved April 4, 2017, from http://world-economic-outlook.findthedata.com/.

International Monetary Fund (IMF). (2017b). *IMF data mapper.* Washington, DC: International Monetary Fund. Retrieved April 4, 2017, from http://www.imf.org/external/datamapper/NGDP_RPCH@WEO/OEMDC/ADVEC/WEOWORLD.

International Monetary Fund (IMF). (2018). *World economic outlook, 2018.* Washington DC: IMF.

International Social Security Association (ISSA). (2018). *Social security programs throughout the world*. Geneva: ISSA.

Investopedia. (2019). *Purchasing power parity (PPP)*. Retrieved February 14, 2019 from https://www.investopedia.com/updates/purchasing-power-parity-ppp/.

Keshavjee, M. (2016). Alternative dispute resolution and its potential or helping Muslim radicals reclaim the higher ethical values underpinning the Sharia. In H. Tiliouine & R. J. Estes (Eds.), *Social progress in Islamic societies: Social, political, economic, and ideological challenges* (pp. 607–622). Dordrecht NL: Springer International Publishers.

Kilmister, M. (2016). *Development in action. Bilateral vs multilateral aid*, October 18. Retrieved April 7, 2017, from http://www.developmentinaction.org/bilateral-vs-multilateral-aid/.

Kinzer, S. (2003). *All the Shah's men: An American coup and the roots of Middle East terrorism*. New York: Wiley.

Krieger, T., & Meierrieks, D. (2011). What causes terrorism? *Public Choice, 147*(1/2), 3–27.

Kurrild-Klitgaard, P., Justesen, M. K., & Klemmensen, R. (2006). The political economy of freedom, democracy and transnational terrorism. *Public Choice, 128*(1/2), 289–315.

Landis, B. (2015). The Islamic world faces its future. *American Diplomacy*, 19–28.

Law, R. (2015). *Routledge history of terrorism*. New York: Routledge Press.

Lozada, C. (2017). *Economic growth is reducing global poverty*. Washington, DC: National Bureau of Economic Research. Retrieved April 1, 2017, from http://www.nber.org/digest/oct02/w8933.html.

Oakes, L., & Gahli, L. (2018). *Ancient Egypt: An illustrated history*. Dayton: Lorenz Monographs.

Organization for Economic Cooperation and Development (OECD). (2015). Net official development assistance by country as a percentage of gross national income in 2015. Retrieved April 15, 2017, from https://data.oecd.org/oda/net-oda.htm.

Organization for Economic Cooperation and Development (OECD). (2016a). *Gross domestic product (in current US dollars)*. Retrieved February 15, 2017, from http://data.worldbank.org/indicator/NY.GDP.PCAP.CD.

Organization for Economic Cooperation and Development (OECD). (2016b). *International development assistance*. Paris: Organization for Economic Cooperation and Development.

Organization for Economic Cooperation and Development (OECD). (2017). *Economy: Developing countries set to account for nearly 60% of world GDP by 2030, according to new estimates*. Paris: Organization for Economic Cooperation and Development.

Organization for Economic Cooperation and Development. (2018). *The 0.7% ODA/GNI target—A history*. Paris: OECD. Retrieved February 20, 2019 from http://www.oecd.org/dac/stats/the07odagnitarget-ahistory.htm.

Organization of Islamic Cooperation. (2018). *Political affairs*. Retrieved February 1, 2019 from https://www.oic-oci.org/dept/?d_id=16&d_ref=11&lan=en.

Pettinger, T. (2013). *Economic impact of migrants and remittances. Helping to simplify economics*. Retrieved February 12, 2017, from http://www.economicshelp.org/blog/6784/economics/economic-impact-of-migrants/.

Piketty, T. (2013). *Capital in the twenty-first century*. (A. Goldhammer, Trans.). Cambridge: Harvard University Press.

Piketty, T. (2015). *The economics of inequality*. (A. Goldhammer, Trans.). Cambridge: Harvard University Press.

Project Open Monograph. (1996). Egyptian violence. *Project Open Monograph*. Retrieved February 1, 2019 from http://www.domini.org/openmonograph/egy9096.htm.

Rahtz, D., & Estes, R. J. (2019). *The universal soldier: The dynamics of gang formation among Jihadist terrorists*. (in preparation).

Richardson, L. (2013). *The roots of terrorism*. London: Routledge.

Rutherford, B. K., & Sowers. (2018). *Modern Egypt: What everyone needs to know*. Oxford: Oxford University Press.

Sehgal, N. (2017). What is foreign direct investment? Personal Finance Guide. Retrieved April 2, 2017, from http://www.fingyan.com/what-is-fd/

Shah, A. (2014). Foreign aid for development assistance. *Global Issues*, September 28, 2014. Retrieved April 1, 2017, from http://www.globalissues.org/article/35/foreign-aid-development-assistance.

Sirgy, M. J., & Estes, R. J. (2018). Understanding Jihadist terrorism in the MENA and Gulf States Region: Quality-of-Life implications for counterterrorism. In L. Lambert (Ed.), *Positive psychology in the Middle East and North Africa: Research, policy, and practice*. Dordrecht: Springer International Publishers.

Sirgy, M. J., Estes, R. J., & Rahtz, D. D. (2018). Combatting jihadist terrorism: A quality-of-life perspective. *Journal of Applied Research in Quality of Life, 13*(4), 813–837.

Sirgy, M. J., Joshanloo, M., & Estes, R. J. (2019). The global challenge of jihadist terrorism: A quality-of-life model. *Social Indicators Research* (1).

Stiglitz, J. (2015). *The great divide: Unequal societies and what we can do about them*. New York: W.W. Norton & Company.

Thompson, D. (2012). The 10 things that economics can tell us about happiness. *Atlantic*. Retrieved May 17, 2017, from https://www.theatlantic.com/business/archive/2012/05/the-10-things-economics-can-tell-us-about-happiness/257947/.

Tiliouine, H., & Estes, R. J. (2016). *Social progress in Islamic societies: Social, political, economic, and ideological challenges*. Dordrecht, NL: Springer International Publishers.

Todaro, M. P., & Smith, S. C. (2012). *Economic development* (11th ed.). New York: Pearson.

Torné, R. (2019). Middle East and North Africa: Overview. *FocusEconomics*, February 11, 2019. Retrieved February 9, 2019 from https://www.focus-economics.com/regions/middle-east-and-north-africa.

United Nations Conference on Trade and Development. (2017). *World investment report, 2017*. Geneva: United Nations Conference on Trade and Development. Annex Table 1. Retrieved July 4, 2017 from http://unctad.org/en/Pages/DIAE/World%20Investment%20Report/Annex-Tables.aspx.

United Nations Department of Economic and Social Affairs. (2017). *Sustainable development knowledge platform*. New York: United Nations Department of Economic and Social Affairs.

United Nations Development Programme. (2017a). *Human development report, 2017: Human development for everyone*. New York: United Nations Development Programme.

United Nations Development Programme. (2017b). *The sustainable development goals*. Retrieved January 10, 2017, from http://www.un.org/sustainabledevelopment/sustainable-development-goals/.

United Nations. (2016). *Arab human development report, 2016*. Retrieved February 1, 2019 from http://arab-hdr.org/

United Nations. (2018). *World population prospects (revised)*. New York: Populations Division.

United States Agency for International Development (USAID). (2007). Foreign direct investment: Putting it to work in developing countries. Retrieved July 2, 2017, from http://pdf.usaid.gov/pdf_docs/Pnadj943.pdf.

Vanham, P. (2015). *5 Trends for the future of economic growth*. Geneva: World Economic Forum. Retrieved July 3, 2017 from https://www.scribd.com/document/307808653/5-Trends-for-the-Future-of-Economic-Growth-Agenda-The-World-Economic-Forum.

Walsh, D. (2019). *El-Sisi may rule Egypt until 2034 under parliamentary plan*. The New York Times, February 14, 2019, A-1. Retrieved February 16, 2019 from https://www.nytimes.com/2019/02/14/world/middleeast/egypt-sisi.html.

World Bank. (2013). World Bank aims to eliminate extreme poverty by 2030. *The Huffington Post*, June 4. Retrieved April 15, 2017, from http://www.huffingtonpost.com/2013/04/02/world-bank-extreme-poverty_n_2999287.html.

World Bank. (2014). *Remittances to developing countries to stay robust this year, despite increased deportations of migrant workers, says WB*. [Press release]. April 11. Retrieved April 15, 2017, from http://www.worldbank.org/en/news/press-release/2014/04/11/remittances-developing-countries-deportations-migrant-workers-wb.

World Bank. (2016). Migration and remittances: Recent developments and outlook. *Migration and Development Brief*, No. 26. Washington, DC: World Bank Group.

World Bank. (2017). *Global economic prospects, 2017: Weak investment in uncertain times*. Washington, DC: World Bank.

World Bank. (2018). *World development report, 2018*. Washington: World Bank.

Worldometers. (2019). *Population of Egypt (2019 and historical)*. Retrieved February 14, 2019 from http://www.worldometers.info/world-population/egypt-population/.

World Population Review. (2018). *The Middle East population, 2019*. Retrieved January 18, 2019 from http://worldpopulationreview.com/continents/the-middle-east-population/.

Chapter 4
Cultural Drivers of Jihadist Terrorism and Increasing Religiosity

Abstract This chapter focuses on cultural and religious factors related to the rise of the Islamist jihadist movement. We make the distinction between the Islamic worldview and ideology and place much of jihadist beliefs that motivate terrorist action in the category of ideology. We discuss the cultural drivers of jihadism couched in the context of religious-cultural paradigms. Specifically, we explore cultural and religious factors that drive the behavior or actions of radical Islamist jihadists toward violence, factors such as grievance and humiliation crisis, revenge and the need to defeat the enemy, establishment of the Islamic State and the re-establishment of the Islamic caliphate, the vanguard of the *ummah*, martyrdom and reward in the afterlife, glorification of Allah, defending sacred places, the temporal paradigm, and chivalric and heroic feats.

Keywords Islamic worldview · Islamic ideology · Muslim grievance · Muslim humiliation · Islamic state · Islamic caliphate · *Ummah* · Martyrdom

4.1 Introduction

The Messenger of Allah, peace and blessings be upon him, said, "You will not enter Paradise until you believe, and you will not believe until you love each other. Shall I show you something that, if you did, you would love each other? Spread peace between yourselves."[1]

First, … these are not suicide operations [Islam forbids suicide.] We are protecting ourselves … The Jews attack and kill our civilians—we will kill their civilians too. … From the first drop of blood [the bomber] spills on the ground, he goes to Paradise. The Jewish victims immediately go to Hell (Frankel, Gellman, & Blumenfeld, 2004).

---

[1] https://abuaminaelias.com/dailyhadithonline/2012/03/16/hadith-on-love-you-will-not-enter-paradise-until-you-love-each-other-for-the-sake-of-allah/.

© Springer Nature Switzerland AG 2019
M. J. Sirgy et al., *Combatting Jihadist Terrorism through Nation-Building*, Human Well-Being Research and Policy Making, https://doi.org/10.1007/978-3-030-17868-0_4

The scholarly review of the topic of terrorism or Islamist jihadi radicalization suggests that it is impossible to identify a comprehensive model to explain the phenomenon of jihadism (Christmann, 2012; el-Aswad, 2016a; Roy, 2007; Spataro, 2008). However, an examination of the socio-cultural environment can allow a better understanding of the more general or cultural drivers that can lead to religious extremism and political violence prompted by Islamist jihadist and radical-dogmatic ideology. This chapter proposes two key theses or concepts. First, the use of the concept of "worldview," including the terms "culture" and "religion," may augment dialogue and enlarge the circles of perspectives that complement, contrast, or go beyond the narrow or strict definition of religious beliefs per se. Second, it is important to draw a distinction between the concept of worldview and that of ideology. As will be subsequently shown, the concept of worldview indicates belief systems and related symbolic actions, while ideology, a subcategory of worldview, implies certain economic and political orientations related particularly to power. The goal here is to highlight the differences between traditional (moderate) Islamic tenets or worldview and those tenets or ideologies embraced by the extremists. These two concepts fit the chapter's main objective seeking to draw a distinction between the Islamist Jihad' ideological-cultural orientation, on the one hand, and the overarching (moderate) Muslim worldviews, on the other. The distinction is crucial for this examination as parts of the terrorists' ideology and mission are assumed by the Islamist jihadists to be related to the worldviews and experience of many Muslims.

In the recent past due to the increasing levels of education, new technology, and ease of travel, Muslim societies have evolved into more open and enlightened in their views of the world. Consequently, in the mainstream Muslim culture religion has become a matter of choice, not just heritage and ritual. Militant Islamist jihadists, however, cling to a narrow and radical view which they try to impose on the rest of the Muslim countries (Rougier, 2007). They use flags, emblems, headbands, graffiti, digital media, social media tags and other symbols to recruit and radicalize moderate Muslims. The militants of global Islamist jihadism use religious or sacred scripts, mainly the Qur'an and the Hadith (tradition and deeds of the Prophet Muhammad), in their attempt to legitimize their ideology and call to arms. They also cite and quote writings of Muslim scholars ('*ulama*') or religious authorities (see Box 4.1), particularly those of Salafi and Wahhabi scholars (see Box 4.2), who serve their ideological goals. It is worth mentioning that individuals, once exposed to particular Islamist jihadi groups, are persuaded that the jihadi organizations are legitimate and credible sources of Islamic interpretation (Wiktorowicz, 2005; Steinback, 2011). Nevertheless, Muslim scholars refute jihadi radical doctrine or ideology describing and dismissing it as erroneous religious innovation (*bid'ah*). "Radicals don't express traditional Islam but try to recast Islam as a militant ideology" (Roy, 2007, p. 57).

Box 4.1: Religious Authorities

The religious authorities here include major schools of thought (*madhāhab*) and jurisprudence. For the Sunnis, there are at least four major schools reflecting different opinions on the laws and obligations of the *shari'a*. These schools include the Shafi'ī, Malikī, Hanafī, and Hanbalī. They are not sects and have no major doctrinal differences; rather, they represent scholarly interpretations and opinions on details of Islamic law and its applications in daily life (el-Aswad, 2012a, p. 157; Center for American Progress, 2011). Other writings include those of Muslim theologians such as Abu al-Hasan Mawardi, Imam al-Nawawi, Abu Hamid al-Ghazali, and Abul Ala Maududi.

Box 4.2: Salafism

The Salafi or Salafism (*Salafiyya*) is a Sunni purist–reform movement calling for a return to Islam as understood and enacted by the pious forefathers or ancestors (*as-salaf aṣ-ṣāliḥ*). The Wahhabi or Wahhabism is a movement within the Sunnis established in Saudi Arabia by Mohammad ibn 'Abd al-Wahhab (1703–1792), which regards the *Qur'an* and *Hadith* as fundamental texts and considers Sufism, mysticism, and Shi'ism as forms of non-orthodox Islam. Wahhabi scholars include Ibn Taymiyya (1263–1328), and Muhammad ibn 'Abd al-Wahhab, among others (el-Aswad, 2012a).

The discussion in this chapter attempts to provide the reader with a better understanding of the insights derived from literature and research on the cultural drivers of jihadism and its use by the Islamist fringe to provide legitimacy to their political agenda, including the justification for the use of terrorism. Although many studies have provided considerable insights on jihadism, there is seems to be a gap in the research (Perry & Howard, 2008). For instance, researchers who blame Islam for its allegedly violent jihad extremism overlook the fact that most ordinary Muslims advocate peace and a peaceful life (el-Aswad, 2003, 2006; Mezzetti, 2017). Other researchers, however, argue that the spread of jihadism among specific Muslim groups, including converts, in different places is caused by cultural drivers such as alienation, ill-being, inequality, and social exclusion in both Muslim and Western societies (Andrews, 2008; Roy, 2007; Zimmerman, 2007). This chapter offers a broad comparative framework of Muslim worldviews and the cultural drivers of the ideology and action of jihadism at both local and global levels. In doing so, we hope that it will contribute a more robust and insightful framing for these past examinations and for future work in the area.

This chapter applies a comparative and multi-method qualitative approach to delineate the most important cultural drivers of Islamist jihadists that cause them to transgress overarching Muslim worldviews and practices. In seeking to provide a comprehensive and wide-ranging examination of this issue, this chapter uses, in addition to a review of scholarly work, information collected from various mass media outlets (such as Al-Jazeera and Al-Arabiya) as well as online archives. This inquiry casts a wide net of media networks and sources to include print news, broadcast news, videos on YouTube, internet websites, cyber forums, livestreaming and other online social media. This broadened and modern concept of media (Taylor, 2007) makes it possible to explore and better evaluate websites of organizations, centers and institutions dealing with Muslim Islamist extremism and jihadism within an integrated analytical framework.

Insofar as this research considers the interaction between the various domains of information and resources, it aims to yield an analysis which can capture the true dynamics of the phenomenon of Islamist jihadism within cultural-ideological and social contexts.

4.2   Muslim Worldviews Versus Islamist Jihadi Ideology

It is important to note at the outset that there is neither Church nor clergy in Islam as is the case in Christianity. This is to say, Muslims emphasize that the relationship between humans and God is direct or without any sort of mediation. Although the exegeses (interpretations of the text) of the religious scholars ('*ulama*') significantly contribute to Islamic tradition and practices, access to sacred texts in Islam is not restricted to scholars or specialists in religious knowledge. (el-Aswad, 2012a). Any person able to read, however basically, has access to scriptures. Sacred scriptures and interpretations of religious doctrines are also accessible on the Internet, allowing people to read, interpret, and discuss religious texts. Put differently, scholars, religious leaders and men of religious learning do not have "a monopoly on sacred authority where Sufi shaykhs, engineers, professors of education, medical doctors, army and militia leaders, and others compete to speak for Islam" (Eickelman & Piscatori, 1996, p. 211). Osama Bin Laden, a civil engineer, established the terrorist group of al-Qaeda (Eickelman, 2002) and presented himself as the defender of Islam and weak people, such as women and children. "Contemporary Islamist jihadists, whether the ISIS or others, have simply picked and chosen different interpretations and precedents and used them as rationalization for their conduct" (Bassiouni, 2016, p. 556). It is worth mentioning that most moderate Muslims disapprove of Islamist terrorist's religious assumptions such as those of Islamists, Al-Qaeda and ISIS (Abou El Fadl, 2005; Warikoo, 2017). It is instructive to refer here to Bruce Lincoln's comparison between the ideologies of George W. Bush and Osama Bin Laden in which he traces a strong convergence of perspective between the two leaders: in dividing the world into two opposing camps of good and evil and using the image of children as innocent victims in justifying their motives and drivers (Lincoln, 2003).

As opposed to ideology, worldview is an interpretative and integrative paradigm encompassing the assumptions through which people view the world in which they live and with which they interact. Worldview is comparable to "Weltanschauung," patterns of thought, perceptual framework, cognitive orientation, and meaning system (Lee, 2004). The main concern here is not merely with the intellectual and cognitive aspects of the worldview but also with the socio-cultural and subjective domains in which individuals locate and define themselves in their relations to others. Worldview, shared by large groups of people, is generated by people's aspiration to reach a unified comprehension of the world, drawing together facts, principles, assumptions, generalizations, and answers to ultimate questions. It constitutes the common understanding that makes possible common practices and a widely shared sense of legitimacy (el-Aswad, 2012a, 2016a).

Though worldview represents a cultural phenomenon, it is different from ideology.

The function of ideology is to make an autonomous politics possible by providing the authoritative concepts that render it meaningful, the persuasive image by means of which it can be sensibly grasped. It is, in fact, precisely at the point at which a political system begins to free itself from the immediate governance of received tradition, from the direct and detailed guidance of religious or philosophical canons on the one hand and from the unreflective precepts of conventional moralism on the other, that formal ideologies tend to emerge and take hold. (Geertz, 1973, pp. 218–19)

Ideology "is essentially linked to the process of sustaining asymmetrical relations of power—that is the process of maintaining domination" (Thompson, 1984, p. 4). Worldviews, contingent on cultural traditions, are clusters of ideas, beliefs, shared meanings or understandings, and practices that render social life possible. Islam is dealt with here as a cultural matrix of the worldviews of ordinary Muslims and not as political ideology. Basic components of Muslim worldview encompass values such as peace, sharing, equality, dignity, belonging, unity, social justice, patience, honor, justice, mercy (*rahmah*), freedom, cosmic capital (not ruthless capitalism), divine livelihood (*rizq*), predestination, ascription of success to God, and doing good deeds as part of worship (el-Aswad, 2012a).

The Arabic word "Islam," meaning both submission to Allah and the maintenance of peaceful relationships with people, is a core concept in Muslim identities and worldviews. Islamist Jihadi extremist groups, however, differ from many Muslims in the sense that they do not advocate peace and tolerance; rather, they advocate and carry out violent actions. Although Islam is based on five pillars, Jihad is sometimes considered the six pillars of Islam (Morgan, 2010). The five pillars of Islam are the testimony of faith (*shahāda*; *there is no god but Allah and Muhammad is His prophet*), praying (*salāt*) five times daily, almsgiving (*zakāt*), fasting (*siyām*) during the month of Ramadan, and participating in the pilgrimage (*hajj*) to Mecca. These five pillars must be observed by ordinary Muslims regardless of their sect, occupation, education, or exegeses of religious scholars or '*ulama*' (el-Aswad, 2012a, p. 11). The meaning or importance of 'jihad' to ordinary Muslims will be discussed subsequently.

By and large, Islamic worldviews encompass major five paradigms: doctrinal, communal, ontological, spatial, and temporal (see Fig. 4.1). First is the doctrinal

Fig. 4.1 Islamic
Worldviews

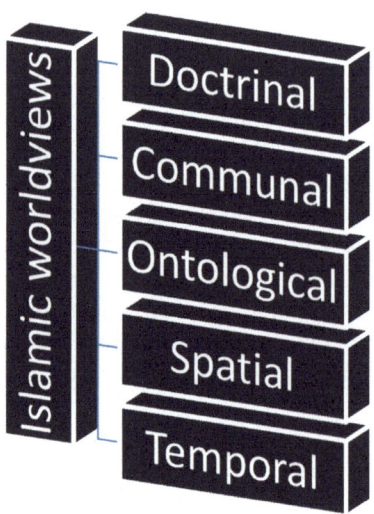

paradigm, where the focus is placed on the way Muslims, in theory and practice, deal with the doctrine of the unity or oneness (*tawḥīd*) of God, implying complete submission to Allah by declaring the religious testimony (*shahāda*), mentioned above. It is to be noted that the first line of the *shahāda* in Arabic (*lā ʾilāha ʾillā allah*) and the seal of Muhammad (*rasūl allah*) are used as the identifying sign or insignia of the flag of the terrorist group of the Islamic State (IS), formerly ISIS (Daesh), or the Islamic State of Iraq and the Levant (ISIL). Second is the communal paradigm, showing the way Muslims relate to each other through the encompassing concept of the ummah, or universal Muslim community. Third is the ontological paradigm, explicating how the world is constructed and how its elements are categorized in term of this world, eschatology (*barzakh*)[2] and the hereafter within broad Muslim frameworks. Fourth is the spatial paradigm, dealing with sacred geographies and sanctified places with which Muslims identify themselves (el-Aswad, 2006, 2012a). The most sacred places are Mecca, the city in which the Ka'ba (*qibla*), the sacred sanctuary and pilgrimage, is located; Medina (historically Yathrib), the city to which the Prophet migrated when he was forced to depart Mecca; and Jerusalem (Al-Quds), the first place (*qibla*) toward which Muslims turned for prayer before the Ka'ba in Mecca. Fifth is the temporal or calendrical paradigm, which regulates Muslims' discursive and non-discursive actions, including beliefs in the limitation of this worldly life and the eternity of the afterlife, rituals, prayers, and other practices (el-Aswad, 2012a).

Politically oriented extremist and militant groups such the Taliban, al-Qaeda, Da'ish or the Islamic State (ISIS), the Islamic State of Iraq and the Levant (ISIL),

---

[2]Eschatology (*barzakh*) is a period of time between death and resurrection, the life beyond the grave, between and betwixt, liminal, mediation, or intermediary between two entities (el-Aswad, 2012a, p. 182).

Al Shabab, and Boko Haram (in Somalia)[3] among others use Islam as a tool justifying their violent actions (el-Aswad, 2016a). The Islamist jihadists use global religious networks not only to spread their extreme mission, but also to compete with the established conventional community of religious scholars (Bunt, 2003). They inspire hate, disgust and contempt toward those who disagree with them. For example, they declare and stigmatize other people including Muslims, who do not accept their radical jihadi ideology, as being apostate (*murtad*) and disbelievers or polytheists (*kafirs*). A mere difference of opinion does not turn a Muslim into a *kafir* or apostate (Bassiouni, 2016). According to Islamic jurisprudence (*fiqh*), the accusation of apostasy or polytheism against Muslims is deemed to be a serious and unforgivable sin (Bassiouni, 2016; Morgan, 2010). The jihadists' attack on Christian and Jewish people (among other non-Muslims) is also a violation of Islamic worldviews. People of the Book, Christians and Jews, are allowed to practice their religion in peace in an Islamic country (Morgan, 2010, p. 183). It is worthy to note that believers in Abrahamic religions as well as adherents of sects within a particular religion co-exist in peace, but ideological and political differences and the lack of constructive dialogue result in grave conflict that negatively affects the well-being of most of Middle East and Muslim countries (el-Aswad, 2019).

Though latent, shared worldviews and beliefs influenced by Muslim tradition have played a decisive role in Muslim countries' socio-political history and have manifested themselves powerfully in critical historical moments. The worldviews of both Muslim intellectuals and common persons, which endow them with a unique imaginative sense of engagement with a transcendent and superior reality, accentuates the theme of a divine, cosmic, invisible higher power surpassing any other. Such a belief represents an inexhaustible source of spiritual and emotional empowerment, which may be in certain critical circumstances become politically mobilized (el-Aswad, 2002, 2003). However, radical Islamist jihadists view and use Islam as a political ideology for achieving their political agenda. "An ideology is a project with a clear blueprint that requires only mechanical implication… Islamism has betrayed many of the tenets of Islam as a divine message; as a way of life; as a civilization, polity, and state; as a religion; and as a body of thought composed of a moral and ethical system" (Rajaee, 2007, p. 4). Put differently, Islamist extremists apply their ideology using religious or Islamic concepts, nevertheless they appeal to the minority, not the majority, of Muslims.

4.3   Cultural Drivers of Islamist Jihadism

This section discusses the cultural drivers of jihadism by comparing the concept of jihad as used by ordinary Muslims, impacted by their religious worldviews with the extreme form of jihad as used by the fanatical Islamist jihadists. Furthermore,

---

[3]Boko Haram's name roughly translates to "Western education is forbidden" (el-Aswad, 2016a, p. 364).

the section addresses the main Islamic cultural paradigms as being held and used differently by ordinary Muslims, on the one hand and the extremist jihadists, on the other.

The Arabic word *jihād*, literally means "struggle," referring to people's spiritual struggle to control animalistic impulses as well as their inner life. The objective of jihad is to attain salvation or liberation through one's own efforts. In other words, the serious effort a person expends toward knowing and controlling her/his inner life is perceived as a spiritual or holy struggle. Jihad is a model of private and public (individual and collective) conduct that should be carried out by faithful Muslims. In this sense, jihad, not restricted to the current meaning of a religiously and politically externalized and mobilized war (el-Aswad, 2012a), signifies an essential drive for Muslim to overcome a physical or worldly self to attain a higher spiritual self.

There is a distinct difference between the ideology of jihadists (Salafi Sunni and Shi'a), and the overarching Islamic worldviews and practices shared by the majority of the Muslims worldwide (el-Aswad, 2012b, 2012c). See Box 4.3. The problem is that people, not educated by or affiliated with formal religious institutions such as Al-Azhar, have been engaged in both extreme religious and political activities. For example, laymen such as Hasan al-Banna, a teacher who founded the Muslim Brotherhood in Egypt, and Sayyid Qutb, a fundamentalist thinker who was not trained as a religious scholar, have become inspiring leaders of many radical and Islamist jihadist groups (Calvert, 2010; el-Aswad, 2012d). Moreover, the radical jihadi ideology is built upon ultra conservative Islamic religious principles, producing a single-minded focus on violent jihad. It is the Jihadi ideologist, such as Sayyid Qutb, who divides the world into the sphere of faithful Muslims versus the sphere of ignorance (*jahiliyya*), including the infidel and apostate that must be resisted and defeated (Abou El Fadl, 2005; Calvert, 2010; el-Aswad, 2012d).

Box 4.3: The Two Traditions of Islam

The Sunni Muslims accept all four caliphs (successors to Muhammed) as being legitimate, including the caliph Ali (Muhammed's son-in-law and cousin). In contrast. Shi'a Muslims reject the first three caliphs before Ali. They regard them as illegitimate successors to Muhammed. The Sunni Muslims treat the prophet Muhammed and the holy Qur'an as final authority. As such, they reject Shi'a succession of the imams. The Shi'a Muslims accept the imams as leaders in both political and religious spheres. In contrast, the Sunni Muslims have a long-standing tradition to separate political and religious leaders. Imams are not accepted as political leaders. The imams have strict authority for Shi'a Muslims. Their pronouncements carry much weight and must be obeyed. They are held on a pedestal and viewed as sinless authorities. They also have the authority to appoint their successors. In contrast, Sunni Muslims do not relegate ultimate authority to the imams (Martin, 2018).

There is always a strong political element in radical Islamist Jihadists' actions including, for example, suicide bombing (Asad, 2007), death threats against intellectuals, kidnapping or hostage taking, and violence against women. Such actions exist outside the worldview or belief system and jihad practices of normative Islam (el-Aswad, 2016a). The radical Islamist jihadists' strategy is to denigrate, isolate, and terminate or destroy any group or anyone who opposes their political goals. Islamist movements that apply the ideology of political Islam are not essentially religious groups concerned with issues of doctrine, beliefs, and faith, but political organizations manipulating Islam to achieve their goals (el-Aswad, 2012a). Moderate Muslim scholars deny that these radical jihadi groups have anything to do with Islam. Islam does not proliferate violence (Brown, 2011; Lee, 2010). Furthermore, some scholars, including the Saudi Grand Mufti say ISIS fighters are harming Islam and Muslims. He claims "that Islamic State (ISIS) jihadists are actually 'Israeli soldiers'" (Arutz Sheva, 2015).

The following is a brief account of the cultural drivers of jihadism couched in the context of religious-cultural paradigms. In other words, we will explore in the sections that follow cultural and religious factors that drive the behavior or actions of radical Islamist jihadists toward violence.

4.3.1 Grievance and Humiliation Crisis

The essential contention of the Islamist jihadist is that the Muslim world is plagued by grievance and sense of injustice, many of which are caused by the West. The roots of the Islamist jihadi violent discourse date back to the second half of the twentieth century, particularly after the defeat suffered in 1948 by the Arab countries against Israel, when nation-states started being viewed as incapable of restoring the dignity of Muslim Arabs (Mezzetti, 2017; Roy, 2007). After the loss of Jerusalem and in response to the injured pride of Muslim Arabs, strong movements of Islamic revival and zealous religiosity swiftly spread in the 1970s and 1980s (Abou El Fadl, 2005).

Most radical jihadist organizations were formed during the Soviet–Afghan War, 1979–1989. To be more specific, the anti-Soviet Afghan jihad in the 1980s gave birth to many radical jihadi organizations bringing together thousands of foreign fighters and jihadists, including volunteers, to safeguard Afghanistan's long-suffering Muslims. Muslim countries suffered economically and politically after the terrorist attack of September 11, 2001 (by Al-Qaeda) and the declaration of global war on terror in which two Muslim countries, Afghanistan and Iraq, were invaded. The US led coalition invading Muslim countries also provoked fierce threats of violence in Indonesia, the world's largest Muslim-majority country. Western media portrayed these reactions as among the most destabilizing in the Muslim world. The Jihad Militia in Indonesia dispatched fighters to battle Christians in the eastern province of Maluku. The jihadists in this province as well as in Indonesia in general were convinced that the United States, Israel, and the Vatican had a direct hand in the Maluku violence (Hefner, 2002). The perceived humiliation of Muslims in conflict zones served as a strong driver for many individuals, men women, to embrace the jihadi ideology (Christmann, 2012; Hoffman, 2008; Khomami, 2018). The driver here was to resist and repudiate the humiliation of the global Muslim community caused by the former Soviet Union, Western Crusaders, and Zionists (Abdullah, 2007). For example, these radical jihadist's propaganda materials included videos showing the executions of western persons (Barr & Herfroy-Mischler, 2017).

4.3.2 Revenge and Defeat the Enemy

Radical Islamist jihadists are driven or motivated by a desire for revenge, particularly in retaliation for losing a loved one or a perceived social injustice. Grievance and psychological distress generate a range of cultural and socio-economic drivers prompting individuals to become radicalized jihadists (Christmann, 2012). Additionally, radical Islamist jihadists focus on defeating insider and outsider enemies. Insider or local enemies include fraudulent political leaders and corrupt governments of Muslim majority countries. For example, Ayman al-Zawahiri, one of Al-Qaeda's founders, argued that fighting against the dishonest and apostate rulers that govern Muslim countries takes precedence over fighting others, including infidel predators, until these rulers are deposed. Doing so is an individual duty incumbent upon (*fard 'ain*) all Muslims (Brown, 2011). Outsider enemies include Western imperialists, Zionists, and nonbelievers (atheist and polytheist). The fact that the United States invaded Iraq in 2003 because of weapons of mass destruction was viewed as a "lie" and hence, proof of morally unjustified Western aggression (Hoeffel, 2014; Wheeler, 2007). The Islamist jihadists, including Bin Laden attacked Western colonialism or neocolonialism and criticized many Arab and Muslim governments for corruption and subordination to Western and Zionists aggression (Brown, 2011). These Islamist jihadists claim that they strengthen the oppressed Muslims against Western oppressors. Revenge also included enslaving and raping non-Muslim women as well as women belonging to certain Muslim factions and sects such as the Shi'a and Yezidi (Otten, 2017).

4.3.3 Establishment of the Islamic State and Re-establishment of the Islamic Caliphate

Politically, the goal of establishing a universal Islamic state or Caliphate, declared by Abu Bakr al-Baghdadi in Iraq in June 2014, constitutes a core driver of the Islamist jihadi activities of ISIS. These radical jihadists reject traditional political concepts of nation-state and national, regional and international institutions such as the Arab League, the Organization of Islamic Cooperation or the United Nations. Rather, jihadists seek to mobilize Muslims across the globe to join the Islamic state or caliphate. The claim of establishing the Islamic state is based on questionable economic and ethical rationalization. For example, ISIS in 2014 managed to accumulate economic resources from extortion, ransoms, money laundering, bank robberies and the sale of stolen antiquities. These activities generated a daily income of $1–3 million, or up to $1.1 billion annually in addition to the $1.5 billion generated from taking over the banks in Mosul and Tikrit reaching $2.6 billion in total (Gaub, 2015). Additionally, women and minors, including foreigners, were recruited to fight along with men. It is estimated that 4761 (13%) of 41,490 foreign citizens who became affiliated with ISIS in Iraq and Syria between April 2013 and June 2018 were women. A further 4640 (12%) were minors. A report from the London-based International Centre for the Study of Radicalization (ICSR) indicated that 850 British citizens became affiliated with ISIS in Iraq and Syria, including 145 women and 50 minors (Khomami, 2018; Isakhan, 2017).

4.3.4 Vanguard of the Ummah

The universal-collective community of Muslims (*ummah*) constitutes a significant component of the worldview through which Muslims identify themselves and view the world or other people with whom they interact. Regardless of their ethnic, cultural, or national backgrounds, Muslim people perceive themselves as being fully part of the *ummah* (el-Aswad, 2012a, 2016a). Jihadists assume the role of the vanguard sustaining and protecting the universal community of Muslims (*ummah*). For the Islamist jihadists, jihad is a religious obligation and a global mission that must be carried out with the intention of expanding Islam and the Islamic *ummah* (Mezzetti, 2017). However, these Islamist jihadists use this value-laden concept to achieve their own political objectives. For instance, Ayman al-Zawahiri, via video, called for Islamist resurgence not only in the West, but also in India (The Guardian, 2014). Moderate Muslims feel insulted by the Islamist jihadists' claim that they locally and globally are the defenders of all Muslims. Moderate Muslims feel belittled that they cannot defend themselves (Baloch, 2017; el-Aswad, 2016b).

4.3.5 Martyrdom and Reward in the Afterlife

Ordinary Muslims view the world not as a machine that can be understood through the scientific paradigm, but as a living reality. Ontologically, the universe is composed of three worlds: this world, the other world or hereafter, and the world of *barzakh* or eschatology. Despite the multiplicity of Muslim worldviews, the most common perspective Muslims have is that the universe has visible and invisible spheres. The unknowable or invisible (*al-ghaib*), known only to Allah, upon which the entire Muslim worldview is built "can be defined as the belief in Allah, His angels, His books and His prophets as well as to such concepts as fate and the hereafter" (el-Aswad, 2012a, p. 12). The martyr (*shahid*) is considered *mujahid* (related to *jihad*, holy war), referring to "the one who dies defending his religion, country, honor, and property" (el-Aswad, 2002, p. 135). Martyrs seek to secure a favorable place in the afterlife or paradise, marrying black-eyed virgins (houris or ḥūrī, sing, ḥuriyah), by claiming that they receive martyrdom (shahāda) as a reward for protecting Muslims and fighting Muslims' enemies. But moderate Muslims recognize that Islam never encourages terrorizing or killing innocent people, Muslim or non-Muslim. Radical Islamist jihadists use verses of the Qur'an out of context to support their martyrdom. It is worth mentioning that although these radical jihadists commit martyrdom by suicide bombings, they refrain from using terms such as suicide and/or suicide bombing, given the fact that such acts are prohibited by Islamic principles. Various verses of the Qur'an confirm that killing, including committing suicide is utterly prohibited. "And do not kill yourselves (or one another). Indeed, Allah is to you ever Merciful" (Qur'an, 4: 29). "And do not kill the soul which Allah has forbidden (to be killed) except by (legal) right. This has He instructed you that you may use reason" (Qur'an, 6: 151).

4.3.6   Glorification of Allah

Radical Islamist jihadists claim that their mission is based on the sentiment of exaltation or glorification of God as represented in the utterance of Allahu akbar ("Allah is the most great") when they commit acts of violence ('ada'u Allah). They also claim that they sacrifice their lives for the sake of God. However, the glorification of God by killing innocent people is a corrupted contradiction in terms. It is worthy to mention that hundreds of millions of Muslims around the world recite the phrase Allahu akbar more than 100 times a day just in their five daily prayers (Ali, 2017). In their daily lives, Muslims use this phrase, indicating that God is omnipotent, omniscient and omnibenevolent, for many purposes on many occasions such as when recognizing a success event, accomplished strength, displayed beauty, or simply a good deed. This means that Allahu akbar is not a chant of violence or warfare. It is not a call to kill others in the name of Islam (Khan, 2017). It is an ostensible contradiction to hear the radical jihadists confirm that they glorify God by chanting Allahu akbar while committing acts of horrific violence. Jihadists believe that fighting for God assures that Allah is empowering their cause. Consequently, Allahu akbar is now associated with terrorism in the minds of many Westerners due to its repeated use by the Islamist jihadists when they engage in acts of brutal and ruthless violence (Hodges, 2018).

4.3.7   Defending Sacred Places

Cultures organize themselves spatially (Bonnemaison, 2005, p. 83) wherein there exists a continuous dialectic between geographical settings and worldviews. The Islamist jihadists assume the role of the vanguard sustaining and protecting Islamic scared places, particularly Jerusalem and those captured and occupied by the Western and Zionist powers. The declaration of Jihad on the alleged American's occupation of Saudi Arabia, the country of the two sacred places, Mecca and Medina, issued in August 1996, was Osama bin Laden's first call to jihad against the United States (Bin Laden, 2008; Bonhomme & Boivin, 2010; Brown 2011). Another example is represented in Ansar Bait al-Maqdis or Ansar Jerusalem (Supporters of Jerusalem), which is a jihadist radical militant group based in Egypt. From 2011 to 2013, Ansar Bait al-Maqdis operated in the Sinai Peninsula and focused its efforts on Egypt and Jordan while being at peace with Israel. The radical jihadist group made attacks against Egyptian army checkpoints as well as against Sinai pipelines exporting gas to Israel. Ansar Bait al-Maqdis changed its name to Wilayat Sinai (Sinai Province) in 2014 after swearing allegiance to the Islamic State of Iraq and the Levant, ISIS (Al-Arabiya, 2016; Al-Jazeera, 2017).

4.3.8   The Temporal Paradigm

Muslim worldviews are structured not only in spatial and ontological terms, but also in temporal paradigms. For instance, the sacred time of prayers intersects with the sacred place, the *Ka'ba*, toward which Muslims turn in prayer. Also, the temporal paradigm intersects with the ontological paradigm including three worlds: this world, the other world, and the world of *barzakh* (the transitional time between them). Muslims believe in the *Mahdi*, a cosmic figure presupposed to be alive though unseen, which is not merely a belief, but rather an ontological entity linked to the structure of the universe. Both Sunni and S*hi'a* believe that the *Mahdi* will appear before Jesus, the redeemer who will restore justice immediately before the apocalypse and the Day of Resurrection or Judgment, *yaum al-qiyāmah* (el-Aswad, 2002, 2012a).[4] For the jihadists, the apocalyptic fight against the Antichrist or *Dajjal* who appears at the end of the world is a timely and critical driver. The radical Islamist jihadists of ISIS believe that there are three enemies, the Antichrist, the Jews, and the new Crusaders all aiming to destroy Muslims, as signs of the end of the world. The radical jihadists, particularly those belonging to ISIS, have used these beliefs to recruit locals and foreigners to join the final battle of the apocalypse, fighting the Antichrist or *Dajjal* and his allies, that is prophesized to take place in and around Jerusalem (McCants, 2015, p. 147).

---

[4]*Shi'a* people, ordinary and intellectuals alike, believe that Arab and Muslim uprisings since 2011, in addition to natural disasters such as the tsunamis that struck different places in the world, are signs of the expected return of *Mahdi*, the *Twelfth* and last *Shi'a* Imam, who is believed to be alive but in concealment (el-Aswad, 2010, 2012a).

4.3.9 Chivalric and Heroic Feats

Radical Islamist jihadists believe that defeating the global and powerful enemies despite insufficient resources is a sign of bravery and commitment backed by the divine power of God, a core element of their ideology. Achieving military victory against the enemies of Islam is consistent with these radical jihadists' key goal, not only of fulfilling the ideals of Islam on earth, but also of showing military strength and chivalry (van Leeuwen & Weggemans, 2018; Screiber, 1978). For instance, the ISIL's military capacity was high controlling, in 2014, 8 million people with 40,000 troops, a ratio of 500 troops per 100,000 inhabitants, compared to the standard of 100–400 troops customarily used to control 100,000 population living in non-conflict zones (Gaub, 2015). Moderate Muslims, however, recognize that acts of violence such as beheading and executing powerless people including women and children as utter savagery, completely devoid of chivalry and heroism. The United Nation (2015) has shown videos confirming mass execution of dozens of people by Daesh (ISIL) in the Anbar province in the most heinous fashion possible.

4.4 Conclusions

Although studies that deal with jihadism and Islamic political thought are extensive, this chapter, by focusing on Muslim worldviews versus radical jihadi ideology, has hopefully provided greater insight concerning the core cultural and religious drivers related to radical Islamist jihadist terrorism. Theoretically, we have drawn a distinction between the concept of worldview and the concept of ideology as a framework to understand the phenomenon of jihadism and its corruption and exploitation by radical Islamists for their own gains.

Further, this examination employed cross-cultural and comparative analyses, to explicate the relationship between the radical jihadists' ideological-cultural drivers and the overarching Muslim worldviews displaying deep and considerable differences between them. In other words, this inquiry has compared the concept of jihad as used by ordinary Muslims, guided by their religious worldviews, with the extreme form of jihad as used by the fanatical Islamist jihadists. This comparative analysis has shed light on the main Islamic cultural paradigms as being held and used differently by ordinary or moderate Muslims, on the one hand and the radical Islamist jihadists, on the other.

What has hopefully become clear to the reader is the conclusion that the radical Islamist jihadists' ideology and violent actions are motivated by a wide and varied range of cultural-religious drivers including: grievance and humiliation crisis, revenge and defeat of internal and external enemies, re-establishment of the Islamic Caliphate, vanguard of the universal Muslim community (*Ummah*), attainment of martyrdom and reward in the hereafter, glorification of Allah, defending sacred places, involvement in the apocalyptic fight against the Antichrist or *Dajjal*, and bearing chivalric and heroic deeds.

Again, this chapter has attempted to show that cultural and ideological drivers are the ultimate driving forces behind the radical jihadists' militant actions at both local, regional, and global levels. Radical jihadists use religious or sacred scripts, mainly the *Qur'an*, the *Hadith* and the exegesis of religious scholars, in their attempt to legitimize their ideology and acts of violence. The authors and the majority of Muslims worldwide believe that these radical jihadists have corrupted and distorted Islamic principles and tenets in their attempt to rationalize and justify their political ideology.

References

Abdullah, D. (2007). How the Zionist colonization of Palestine radicalized British Muslims. In T. Abbas (Ed.), *Islamic political radicalism: A European perspective*. (pp. 117–130). Edinburgh University Press

Abou El Fadl, K. (2005). *The great theft: Wrestling Islam from the extremists*. New York, NY: Harper San Francisco.

Al-Arabiya (2016). *ISIS brings Egypt and Israel even closer*. Retrieved from https://english.alarabiya.net/en/views/news/middle-east/2016/08/11/ISIS-brings-Egypt-and-Israel-even-closer.html.

Ali, W. (2017). I Want 'Allah Akbar' Back. *The New York Times*. Retrieved from https://www.nytimes.com/2017/11/01/opinion/manhattan-truck-attack-akbar-terrorism.html.

Al-Jazeera (2017). *The silence in Sinai: Covering Egypt's 'war on terror' (Video)*. Retrieved from https://www.youtube.com/watch?v=_kgX-t6Ryic.

Andrews, J. (2008). Sociology of Jihad: How rational people commit atrocities. *The Counter Terrorist, 1*(2), 26–30.

Arutz Sheva (2015). *Saudi Grand Mufti says ISIS are 'Israeli soldiers'*. Retrieved from http://www.israelnationalnews.com/News/News.aspx/205570.

Asad, T. (2007). *On suicide bombing*. New York: Columbia University Press.

Barr, A., & Herfroy-Mischler, A. (2017). ISIL's execution videos: Audience segmentation and terrorist communication in the digital age. *Studies in Conflict & Terrorism*, https://doi.org/10.1080/1057610x.2017.1361282. Retrieved from http://dx.doi.org/10.1080/1057610X.2017.1361282.

Baloch, M. (2017). An Islam that rejects Islamist: The case of Baloch. In R. L. Benkin (Ed.), *What is moderate Islam?* (pp. 97–126). Lanham: Lexington Books.

Bassiouni, C. M. (2016). Islam and contemporary radicalized violence: A historic turning point. In R. J. Estes & H. Tiliouine (Eds.), *Social progress in Islamic societies: Social, political, economic, and ideological challenges* (pp. 547–573). Dordrecht NL: Springer.

Bin Laden, O. (2008). Declaration of jihad against Jews and Crusaders. In M. Perry & E. N. Howard (Eds.), *The theory and practice of Islamic terrorism: An anthology* (pp. 41–48). New York: Palgrave Macmillan.

Bonhomme, B., & Boivin, C. (2010). Osama bin Laden's Declaration of Jihad against Americans: Full Text and Document Analysis. *Milestone Documents in World History*. Retrieved from https://salempress.com/store/pdfs/bin_laden.pdf.

Bonnemaison, J. (2005). *Culture and space: Conceiving a new geography*. London: I.B. Tauris.

Brown, V. (2011). Classical and global jihad Al-Qa'ida's franchising frustrations. In Assaf Moghadam & Brian Fishman (Eds.), *Fault lines in global jihad: Organization, strategic, and ideological Fissures* (pp. 88–116). London: Routledge.

Bunt, G. R. (2003). *Islam in the digital age: E-Jihad, online fatwas and cyber Islamic environments.* London: Pluto Press.

Calvert, J. (2010). *Sayyid Qutb and the origins of radial Islamism.* New York: Columbia University Press.

Center for American Progress. (2011). *Understanding Sharia Law.* Retrieved from https://www.americanprogress.org/issues/religion/reports/2011/03/31/9175/understanding-sharia-law/.

Christmann, K. (2012) *Preventing religious radicalization and violent extremism. A systematic review of the research evidence.* Youth Justice Board. Retrieved from https://www.gov.uk/government/publications/preventing-religious-radicalisation-and-violent-extremism.

Eickelman, D. F., & Piscatori, J. (1996). *Muslim politics.* Princeton, NJ: Princeton University Press.

Eickelman, D. F. (2002). The Arab "street" and the Middle East's democracy deficit. *Naval War College Review, 1*(4), 39–48.

el-Aswad, el-S. (2002). *Religion and folk cosmology: Scenarios of the visible and invisible in Rural Egypt.* Westport, CT: Praeger Press.

el-Aswad, el-S. (2003). Sanctified cosmology: Maintaining Muslim identity with globalism. *Journal of Social Affairs, 24*(80), 65–94.

el-Aswad, el-S. (2006). Spiritual genealogy: Sufism and saintly places in the Nile Delta. *International Journal of Middle East Studies, 38*(4), 501–518.

el-Aswad, el-S. (2010). The perceptibility of the invisible cosmology: Religious rituals and embodied spirituality among the Bahraini Shi'a. *Anthropology of the Middle East, 5*(2), 59–76.

el-Aswad, el-S. (2012a). *Muslim worldviews and everyday lives.* Lanham, MD: AltaMira Press, Rowman & Littlefield Publisher.

el-Aswad, el-S. (2012b). Shia: 1920 to present: Middle East. In A. Stanton, E. Ramsamy, P. Seybolt, & C. Elliott (Eds.), *Cultural sociology of the Middle East, Asia, & Africa: An encyclopedia.* (pp. 1354–1356). Thousand Oaks, CA: SAGE Publications, Inc.

el-Aswad, el-S. (2012c). Sunni: 1920 to present: Middle East. In A. Stanton, E. Ramsamy, P. Seybolt, & C. Elliott (Eds.), *Cultural sociology of the Middle East, Asia, & Africa: An encyclopedia.* (pp. 1360–1361). Thousand Oaks, CA: SAGE Publications, Inc.

el-Aswad, el-S. (2012d). Review of Sayyid Qutb and the origins of radial Islamism. *Digest of Middle East Studies, 21*(1), 267–269

el-Aswad, el-S. (2013). Images of Muslims in Western scholarship and media after 9/11. *Digest of Middle East Studies* (DOMES), *22*(1), 39–56.

el-Aswad, el-S. (2015). Islamic worldview and Islamist ideology: The predicament of sanctity and power. *Papers presented at 114th American Anthropological Association Annual Meeting*: Denver, CO Nov. (pp. 18–22).

el-Aswad, el-S. (2016a). Political challenges confronting the Islamic world. In H. Tiliouine & R. J. Estes (Eds.), *The state of social progress of Islamic societies: Social, economic, political, and ideological challenges.* (pp. 361–377). AG Switzerland: Springer International Publishing.

el-Aswad, el-S. (2016b). State, nation and Islamism in contemporary Egypt: An anthropological perspective. *Urban Anthropology, 45*(1–2), 63–92.

el-Aswad, el-S. (2017). Islamic care and counseling. In Leeming, D.A. (Ed.), *Encyclopedia of psychology and religion* (pp. 1–14). GmbH, Germany: Springer.

el-Aswad, el-S. (2019). *The quality of life and policy issues among the Middle East and North African countries.* New York: Springer.

Frankel, G., Gellman, B., & Blumenfeld, L. (2004). Sheik Ahmed Yassin, Founder of Hamas. *Washington Post,* March 22, 2004.

Gaub, F. (2015). Can ISIL be copied. *European Union Institute for Security Studies, 1*(4), 1–4.

Geertz, C. (1973). *The Interpretation of Cultures.* New York: Basic.

Global Security Org. (2018). *Ansar Bayt al-Maqdis, Wilayat Sinai.* Retrieved from https://www.globalsecurity.org/military/world/para/abm.htm.

Hefner, R. W. (2002). Global violence and Indonesian Muslim politics. *American Anthropologist, 104*(3), 754–765.

Hodges, A. (2018, August 1). Reclaiming 'Allahu Akbar' from semantic pejoration. *Anthropology News Website*. Retrieved from http://www.anthropology-news.org/index.php/2018/08/01/reclaiming-allahu-akbar-from-semantic-pejoration/.

Hoeffel, J. M. (2014). *The Iraq lie: How the White House sold the war*. San Diego, California: Progressive Press.

Hoffman, B. (2008). Al Qaeda resurgent. In M. Perry & E. N. Howard (Eds.), *The theory and practice of Islamic terrorism: An anthology* (pp. 101–112). New York: Palgrave Macmillan.

Isakhan, B. (2017). The Islamic State attacks on Shia holy sites and the "Shrine Protection Narrative": Threats to sacred space as a mobilization frame. *Terrorism and Political Violence*. Retrieved from https://doi.org/10.1080/09546553.2017.1398741.

Khan, A. M. (2017). Reclaiming 'Allahu akbar' from its misuse by terrorists. *Los Angeles Times*. Retrieved from http://www.latimes.com/opinion/readersreact/la-ol-le-new-york-attack-allahu-akbar-20171101-story.html.

Khomami, N. (2018). Number of women and children who joined ISIS significantly underestimated. *The Guardian*. Retrieved from https://www.theguardian.com/world/2018/jul/23/number-of-women-and-children-joining-isis-significantly-underestimated.

Lee, R. D. (2010). *Religion and politics in the Middle East: Identity, ideology, institutions, and attitudes*. Boulder, CO: Westview.

Lee, S. (2004). Constructing an aesthetic Weltanschauung: Freud, James, and Ricoeur. *Journal of Religion and Health, 43*(4), 273–290.

Lincoln, B. (2003). *Holy terrors: Thinking about religion after September 11*. Chicago: University of Chicago Press.

Martin, G. (2018). *Understanding terrorism: Challenges, perspectives, and issues* (6th ed.). Los Angeles: Sage Publications.

McCants, W. F. (2015). *The ISIS apocalypse: The history, strategy, and doomsday vision of the Islamic State*. New York: St. Martin's Press.

Mezzetti, G. (2017). Contemporary Jihadism: A generational phenomenon. *Fondazione ISMU*. Retrieved from http://www.ismu.org/wp-content/uploads/2017/07/Mezzetti_Paper_Jihadism_July2017.pdf.

Morgan, D. (2010). *Essential Islam: A comprehensive guide to belief and practice*. Santa Barbara, California: Praeger/ABC-CLIO.

Otten, C. (2017). *With Ash on their faces: Yezidi women and the Islamic State*. Toronto, ON: Between the Line.

Perry, M., & Howard, E. N. (2008). *The theory and practice of Islamic terrorism: An anthology*. New York: Palgrave Macmillan.

Rajaee, F. (2007). *Islamism and modernism: The changing discourse in Iran*. Austin: University of Texas Press.

Rougier, B. (2007). *Everyday Jihad: The rise of militant Islam among Palestinians in Lebanon* (P. Ghazaleh, Trans.). Cambridge, MA: Harvard University Press.

Roy, O. (2004). *Globalized Islam: The search for a new Ummah*. New York: Columbia University Press.

Roy, O. (2007). The Islamic terrorist radicalization in Europe. In S. Amghhar, A. Boubekeur, & M. Emerson (Eds.), *European Islam: Challenges for society and public policy* (pp. 52–60). Brussels: Center for European Policy Study.

Screiber, J. (1978). *The ultimate weapon: Terrorists and world order*. New York: Morrow.

Spataro, A. (2008). Why do people become terrorists? A prosecutor's experiences. *Journal of International Criminal Justice, 6*, 507–524.

Steinback, R. (2011). Jihad against Islam. *Southern Poverty Law Center* (142). Retrieved from https://www.splcenter.org/fighting-hate/intelligence-report/2011/jihad-against-islam.

Taylor, C. (2007). *A secular age*. Cambridge, MA: Belknap Press of Harvard University.

The Guardian. (2014). *Al-Qaida leader Ayman al-Zawahiri calls for Islamist resurgence in India—video*. Retrieved from https://www.theguardian.com/world/video/2014/sep/04/al-qaida-leader-ayman-al-zawahiri-islamist-india-video.

Thompson, J. B. (1984). *Studies in the theory of ideology*. Berkeley: University of California Press.
van Leeuwen, L., & Weggemans, D. (2018). Characteristics of jihadist terrorist leaders: A quantitative approach. *Perspectives on Terrorism, 12*(4), 55–67.
Warikoo, K. (2017). Islamist extremism: Threat to world peace and security. In R. L. Benkin (Ed.), *What is moderate Islam?* (pp. 25–54). Lanham: Lexington Books.
Wheeler, M. (2007). *Anatomy of deceit: How the Bush administration used the media to sell the Iraq war and out a spy*. Berkley, California: Waster Books.
Wiktorowicz, Q. (2005). *Radical Islam rising: Muslim extremism in the West*. Lanham, Md.: Rowman & Littlefield.
United Nation. (2015). UN confirms mass execution of dozens by Daesh (ISIL) in Anbar province. Retrieved from https://www.youtube.com/watch?v=pIio12t8mRY.
Zimmerman, J. C. (2007). Jihad, theory and practice: A review essay. *Terrorism and Political Violence, 19*(2), 279–288.

Chapter 5
Political Drivers of Islamist Jihad

Abstract Are the political actions of authoritarian regimes—tribal and exclusion-ary—in the MENA region associated with Islamist jihadist terrorist actions? This is the question we will be addressing in this chapter. We do this by describing the history of authoritarian regimes of Libya, Egypt, Syria, Iraq, Saudi Arabia, and Sudan and jihadist terrorist incidents in these countries. We conclude by referring to Tunisia, a country that experienced authoritarian rule but emerged from this experience with democratic bearings. Are there lessons to be learned from the Tunisian experiment in democracy?

Keywords Authoritarian regimes · Democracy · Jihadist terrorism · Islamists

5.1 Introduction

> To achieve a lasting peace in the Middle East takes guts, not guns.
>
> Queen Rania of Jordan[1]

A host of authors and organizations have examined the political nature of the Middle East over the past decades. The political discourse will often reach back to the times of Western and/or Ottoman Empire Occupation of the Middle East and offer interpretations built around such political dynamics as the imposition of political boundaries based on geographic coordinates and not historical tribal and cultural relationships. (cf. Kamrava, 2013) Some authors have offered that such conditions and Western interventions in the regions lead to governmental and political power coalitions which can often lead to authoritarian regime (e.g. Yom, 2016). Other authors (e.g. Bellin, 2004, 2012) looked at the continued survival of these authoritarian regimes across a host of regional and global events. Recent events, the Arab Spring in the region, prompted hopeful predictions for possible future regional political scenarios built

---

[1] https://www.brainyquote.com/quotes/queen_rania_of_jordan_513351.

© Springer Nature Switzerland AG 2019   95
M. J. Sirgy et al., *Combatting Jihadist Terrorism through
Nation-Building*, Human Well-Being Research and Policy Making,
https://doi.org/10.1007/978-3-030-17868-0_5

Table 5.1 Jihadist organizations worldwide and their activity profile

Jihadist organization	Constituency	Adversary
Palestinian Islamic Jihad	Palestinian Muslims	Israel
Hamas	Palestinian Muslims	Israel
Al-Qaeda	Faithful Muslims	Secular governments, nonbelievers, the West
Abu Sayyaf	Filipino Muslims	Filipino government, Western influence
Laskar Jihad	Moluccan Muslims	Moluccan Christians
Jammu-Kashmir groups	Jammu-Kashmir Muslims	India
Algerian/North African cells	Algerian Muslims and Muslims worldwide	Secular Algerian government, the West
Boko Haram	West African Muslims	Nigerian and West African nonbelievers, the West
Islamic State of Iraq and Syria (ISIS) or the Levant	Levant Sunnis	Secular Arab nations, Shi'a, nonbelievers

Source Adapted from Martin (2018, p. 150)

around previous historical culturally linked societies (Stansfield, 2013). Freedom House,[2] an independent Watchdog group that monitors the world's nations for conditions based around freedom and democratic institutions has continually ranked many MENA countries authoritarian. This chapter explores the linkages of political authoritarianism to Islamist jihadi terrorism. See Table 5.1 for a partial list of jihadist organizations worldwide.

We ask the following question in particular: Are the political actions of authoritarian regimes—tribal and exclusionary—in the MENA region associated with jihadist terrorist actions? We explore this question by using an historical assessment of six regimes that are often characterized by Freedom House and others as authoritarian. These are: Libya, Egypt, Syria, Iraq, Saudi Arabia, and Sudan. In the following sections of this chapter we offer a review of recent Islamist jihadist terrorist incidents in these countries. We end our examination with an additional quick review of Tunisia, a country that experienced authoritarian rule, but recently emerged from this experience with democratic bearings. Are there lessons to be learned from the Tunisian experiment in democracy and applied in a wider context to the broader MENA region?

In Chap. 1 of this book we briefly discussed the role of political factors in the experience of anger and frustration among the aggrieved. Specifically, we discussed how authoritarian, tribal, and exclusionary regimes seem to be associated with radicalism and militancy. Many of the political regimes in the MENA region are authoritarian and suppressive of many freedoms that Westerners take for granted (Bellin, 2012). Such regimes tend to be single tribal restricting widespread plural political participa-

---

[2]https://freedomhouse.org.

tion. Those who perceive that their political rights are violated also believe that social change can be brought about only through violent means (Boix, 2011; Crenshaw, 2011). Let us be more specific with examples from our six countries (Dalacoura, 2012; Pargeter, 2009). See Box 5.1.

Box 5.1: Rise of Islamist Extremism May be Related to Political Suppression
The discrediting of leftist ideologies within the Muslim world, like the earlier loss of respect for Nasserite pan-Arabism … has … meant that political Islam has become the main vehicle there for expression … of strongly held dissent. A young man in a Muslim country who wants to make a forceful statement against the existing order has few avenues for doing so except through membership in a radical Islamic group (Pillar, 2001, pp. 45–46).

5.2 Libya

Libya has a long history of marginalizing segments of their society from political participation in governance (Sawani, 2012). Libya has been a Muslim country since the advent of Islam in the MENA region. The oil rich country in North African has only around six million inhabitants. The vast majority of Libyans are members of the dominant Sunni sect. Attempts at spreading Shi'ism in the early parts of the spread of Islam failed to take root in Libya. Attempts to bring in other Muslim sects such as Sufism also proved to be difficult. Muammar Qadhafi had been Libya's leader for over 40 years before being overthrown and killed in 2011. Prior to his overthrow, Colonel Muammar Qadhafi also managed to maintain the religious suppression of Islamist orientations (fundamentalists and jihadists). However, the fall of the Qadhafi regime unleashed ideological forces with contrasting views of Islam. Since then, Libyans have failed to hold on to their moderate Islam and has increasingly been subject to political conflict driven by Islamist religious extremism. The fall of the Qadhafi regime has led to a different form of political authority, namely "Tribalism." Tribalism was a fact of life during the regimes of King Idriss (who was overthrown by Qadhafi) and Qadhafi. The regime of King Idriss relied heavily on tribal alliances to provide political and legal legitimacy for the regime. However, Qadhafi maintained tribal alliances through military coercion. Tribes that were out of line suffered the wrath of the military establishment. The fall of Qadhafi paved way to extreme tribalism and factionalism to be reborn. Libya has turned into a federal state in which different regions asserted their tribal authority over the state, a political structure that existed prior to 1963. The tribal structure did not work in parallel with the modern institutions of the state and central bureaucracy. This failure was an important factor in the disintegration of civil society—civil society requires the existence of civic culture and citizenship. The Islamist movement in Libya today (e.g., Salafists and the Muslim Brotherhood) does not support democracy; they simply tolerate it as long as it does not clash with the primacy of Islamic *sharia* as manifested in Libyan laws. The Islamist movement fiercely denigrates the call for secularism. Islamist forces are now more organized than ever. Islamists have been making significant inroads to establish their political presence in Libya in an attempt to replace the current regime. Consider the following decree from sheikh Salim al-Shaykhi regarding the political program of the Muslim Brotherhood:

> Libya [sic] is a Muslim people, and the religion of Libya is Islam. The Islamist movement is the movement that desires to preserve the Islamic nature of the state through: reinforcing the Islamic character of the state in the sense that people say: 'We are Muslims and it is incumbent to rule and judge according to our religion in our political, economic and social issues. Religion is not [simply a matter of] prayers and ritual worship alone; religion is economics … [and] the political dimension: Islam is a religion that is based upon *sharia* and multiplicity/pluralism (*ta'addudiyah*)'. The ruler does not have any absolute power/authority. (al-Dali, 2011, pp. 6–7)

Liberals in Libya have issued a call of alarm regarding democracy in Libya. Additionally, they and other secular camps have criticized Islamists for wanting to overturn the democratic system of government once they are in a position to rule. To counter the liberals, the extremists among Islamists (e.g., Islamic Movement for Change, IMC or al-Harakah al-Islamiyah li-l-Taghyir) have resorted to a strategy that includes political assassinations. To this day, Islamists in Libya have fought hard against public freedoms, freedom of women, freedom of opinion and expression, freedom to form political parties and associations, as well as freedom to practice religion. Their position is these freedoms must be tightly restricted based on a strict interpretation of Islamic *sharia*.

To counter the Islamist movement in Libya, especially the extremist among them, liberal, nationalist and secularist parties have managed to prop up the current secular institutions, so far (Toaldo, 2016). The outside interventions to support these endeavors can be seen as tenuous.

The liberal and nationalist parties' express loyalty to liberal democracy (Boduszyński, 2015). Some of these parties emerged from opposition to Qadhafi abroad since the early 1980s. Others have long been in the Qadhafi camp. There are also new parties emerging such as the Libyan Democratic Gathering that advocates liberal democracy and human rights. Sawani (2012, p. 21) warns us.

> Observers of activities connected to the founding of political parties can attest to the vagueness or lack of clarity in the many attempts and the inability to formulate clearly defined political programmes. They also lack clear-cut political identity and positions towards current issues. Apparently, an increase in political parties with no ability to play any effective role in political life in the short-term will be witnessed. It is important, however, to stress the warning issued by the newly set up Libyan Democratic Association regarding the campaign by forces that use mosques as well as billboard and posters in public places to wage war on the work of political parties. There is no doubt that such antipathy to political parties may constitute a threat to democratic life and limit the scope of freedom of opinion and expression.

Islamic State (ISIS) fighters established their first base in Libya outside of Syria and Iraq in 2014. News reports indicate that Islamic State militants in Libya supported terrorist operations in Europe in 2017. Although they are losing ground in Libya due to support from Egypt, Qatar, and the US, they remain a major threat to Libya's stability. The forecast is that the Islamist jihadists are likely to retain some semblance of control and will continue to be a significant challenge in the near future (The American Foreign Policy Council's World Almanac of Islamism, 2018).

To counter the Islamist jihadist movement in Libya, the challenge is not only in propping up liberal, nationalist, and secularist parties, but also to change Libyans' sentiment away from the dominance of the state. Doing so could lead to a culture of democracy. A cultural environment that can pave way to true democracy itself (Obeidi, 2008, p. 16). That is, Libyans have to free their minds from the shackles of state oppression (the memories of the oppressive Qadhafi regime) and begin to express themselves freely in accordance with democratic rules of governance such as elections and referenda.

5.3 Egypt

Nineteen seventy-eight was a watershed moment in the Middle East. To understand what has transpired in Egypt (and for that matter MENA) we do need to go back to that year. It was that year, 1978, when President Anwar Sadat made peace with Israel. The peace treaty caused a great upheaval and schism in Egyptian society because it was opposed by many Muslims in the MENA region. Sadat's peace overtures focused strictly on a peace treaty between Egypt and Israel. Governments and rulers of the Arab states expected a comprehensive peace settlement as a solution to the Arab-Israeli conflict that included the return of the Sinai Desert to Egypt, the West Bank to Jordan, the Golan Heights to Syria, and a resolution of the Palestinian problem. Islamists in Egypt were outraged by the peace treaty. Three years later in 1981, Islamist extremists assassinated President Sadat in a large part due to the peace treaty with Israel. Sadat's vice-president was Hosni Mubarak who took over the government's reigns after the assassination.

Mubarak managed to build and preserve an authoritarian rule on the country for three decades (Shehata, 2009). The authoritarian nature of his regime became progressively more authoritarian over the years. Mubarak consolidated his political power under the presidency, and his control over the ruling party, the National Democratic Party. His regime clamped down on opposition parties using a variety of means such as controlling the news media and other information and publication venues. Laws were passed and often strictly enforced against any criticism of the presidency and the ruling party; thus, freedom of the press was severely restricted. Freedom of assembly was also severely restricted. A wide mix of basic rights were violated under the guise of the Emergency Law (in force since 1981). The use of torture became a tool to be applied in the suppression of political dissent.

This political repression led to the rise of several Islamist militant groups such as al-Gama'a al-Islamiyya and al-Jihad al-Islami. Violence erupted, and Egypt became engulfed in violence between 1992 and 1997. By 1998, state actions aimed at repressing the threat to the government had managed to severely hamper (if not eliminate) these Islamist militant groups. Opposition to the regime re-emerged in the mid-2000s; however, the new rise of opposition was not led by Islamist groups, but mostly by a broader and more mainstream Egyptian civil society. In 2005–2006, a broad coalition of opposition activists, called Kifaya (Enough) organized street demonstrations to block Mubarak's son from transitioning into the presidency. The Kifaya movement paved way to a greater democracy movement in Egypt exemplified in the growing independence of the judiciary, labor unions and other professional organizations challenging the government's economic policies through wildcat strikes and street demonstration, etc. Prompted and inspired by the success of Tunisia's revolt against their country's rulers, Egyptians in 2011 demonstrated in greater frequency with the seemingly clear purpose of toppling the president. The government tried to quell these demonstrations, but to no avail. Government attempts (at times, viewed by the population as increasingly violent) to quell the demonstrations caused a nation-wide revulsion. This, in turn, caused further mass demonstration, which finally convinced Mubarak to step down.

In the aftermath of Mubarak stepping down, the army took control of the government and began to the process to institute constitutional and social reforms. However, the Supreme Council of the Armed Forces made decisions that were perceived by the public as lacking in substantive reforms. The changes that were made were viewed as merely cosmetic in the sense that the street revolution managed to topple a few high-level officials of the old guard. Protesters again took to the streets in large numbers and in the ensuing confrontations the ruling generals were compelled to make more substantive actions. These actions included the arrests of dozens of high-level government officials including Mubarak himself.

In the weeks and months that followed new elections allowed the Muslim Brotherhood to reassert itself in political life and civil society. The group gained political legitimacy and through democratic elections secured a great deal of new-found political power. In 2012, Mohammed Morsi of the Muslim Brotherhood took over as president. Morsi moved quickly in making several key changes in government including ousting many top army officers and replacing them with officials that he considered trustworthy and supportive of his presidency. These moves were viewed by many as a direct threat to the autonomy of Egypt's armed forces, and the Supreme Council of Armed Forces. A coalition of liberal, nationalist, and secular groups also became quick concerned with the rise to power of the Muslim Brotherhood and Morsi's moves to consolidate their power in the Egyptian government's institutions and political environment. This concern from this more liberal and secular coalition regarding the actions and future intent of the Muslim Brotherhood caused a major schism in the Egyptian society.

The Supreme Council of Armed Forces felt compelled to intervene again to restore order. It did so by moving against those who had gained power, that is the Muslim Brotherhood. The subsequent arrests and imprisonments for many of them forced their cadres to go underground again. President Morsi was ousted, arrested, convicted, and sentenced to prison. The Supreme Council of the Armed Forces assumed control of the government again. In 2013, Army chief Abdul Fattah al-Sissi assumed the presidency. In 2014, Islamist extremists intensified their insurgency in the Sinai Peninsula, and the insurgency continues today.

Authoritarian rule, tribalism, and political exclusion remains today and is deeply entrenched in Egyptian society. In 2018, al-Sissi appointed a new minister of defense and the country's prime minister bypassing ratification from both the Supreme Council of the Armed Forces and Egypt's parliament—the two institutions that provide checks and balances. These two institutions have seemed to have forfeited their political rights paving way to authoritarian rule. Again, the current form of an authoritarian rule seems destined to be in place for the foreseeable future. Sissi is repeating history by systematically removing obstacles to his power (Goldberg, 2018). More recently, the New York Times reported that Egypt's parliament has cleared way for El-Sisi to rule until 2034 (Walsh, 2019). What are the chances that Islamist militancy will rise again? The authors feel that is a very real possibility and one that may occur sooner rather than later.

5.4 Syria

As with our previous discussion on Egypt, there is an apparent starting point to help understand the current situation in Syria. To best capture the discussion of authoritarian rule in Syria we must go back to 1971 when Hafiz al-Assad became president (Encyclopedia Britannica, 2018). The Assad regime, for the most part, was one of brutality for anyone who opposed or gave any indications of dissent. His government had no hesitation to use violent means to suppress political opposition. The police, military, and paramilitary forces were sent by Assad against any group or individual voicing opposition. There was hope when the current president, Bashar al-Assad, inherited the presidency following his father's death in 2000. Much of the country perceived him as a modernizer and a reformer. Syrians had high hopes that his regime would be more democratic and less authoritarian. Bahar al-Assad promised wide-ranging reforms across all the sectors of society. These included economic reforms, social reforms, political reforms, etc. In an environment of hoped for dialogue and change, pro-democracy groups demanded an end to the authoritarian practices of the Assad regime. While Bashar flirted with some reforms, these reform overtures were short-lived. The new Assad government responded in the same manner of the old government of his father. The practice of surveillance of opposition groups, torture of suspected subversives, and brutal violence leveled against anyone who spoke ill of the regime was resurrected and persecuted with vigor. The population continued to seek resolution of the many economic, social, and political ills and grievances to that had plagued Syria. Wealth distribution was extremely skewed. Only a small handful of connected families seem to control much of the wealth in the country. Most Syrians were trapped in dire poverty. Natural disasters also arrived to contribute to the misery and pain of the population. The country experienced the worst drought in the country's modern history causing increasingly widespread poverty in the rural areas; this poverty, in turn, drove many rural families to migrate to the large cities, settling in shantytowns. The country was ripe for rising protests and violent opposition to take hold.

The first major protests took place in 2001 in the drought-stricken rural province of *Dar'a*. These protests were quelled by security forces who used harsh means—mass arrests and lethal weapons firing on demonstrators. Videos of these protests and the brutal response from the government's security forces went viral causing widespread popular dissension. Religious affiliations also fed the dissent and anger. Most of the members of the government security forces were from the Alawite sect (a Muslim sect, different from the Sunni sect). In contrast, most of the protesters were mostly Sunnis. This situation caused a great deal of friction between Alawites and Sunnis in greater Syria.

Over time, the protests increased in strength and size. The Assad regime repeatedly responded brutally with military strikes—tanks, artillery, and helicopter strikes causing many civilian casualties. Meanwhile, opposition militias continued gaining momentum in 2011, and by 2012 the country was ravaged by a full-fledged civil war. The harsh government response against militia opposition groups and civilian casualties initiated a mass migration of civilians into safer areas including migration to neighboring countries (Turkey, Lebanon, Jordan, and Iraq) and other European countries.

Beginning in the summer of 2011, the United States, European allies, as well as the Arab League demanded Bashar al-Assad to step down and allow democracy to take hold. When he refused sanctions followed—targeting senior members of the Assad regime. Assad continued to receive aid and unfettered support through this time from Iran, Russia, China, and the Hezbollah faction of Lebanon. A support that also included military and intelligence aid to prop up the regime. Two of these supporters also happened to hold permanent seats on the UN Security Council. A fact that limited a UN role in seeking peace in Syria. Little changed, and the opposition militia forces and their supporters suffered even more brutal attacks.

In 2013, the Assad regime was blamed for a chemical weapons attack in the Ghouta suburbs of Damascus. Hundreds of civilians died or were horribly injured. The US, UK, and France blamed the regime; the regime blamed the rebel fighters. In 2014, the Western Alliance accepted an agreement worked out with the Russian supporters of Assad that compelled the regime to destroy its arsenal of chemical weapons. In the same year, Assad ran for a third term and won by 88.7% of the votes. These votes were cast in areas of the country under the regime's control; and as such, the Western Alliance declared the vote was a farce.

In same period of these events, Syria witnessed the major surge of the Islamic State which managed to overrun large swathes of territory in Syria and Iraq. Russia came to the rescue of Assad in the first half of 2015. The Russians started to conduct a major campaign against all rebel factions that also included Islamic State (ISIS) militants. Russian air strikes (most done without advanced "smart bombs" that allow more precise targeting) against the various rebel factions created a great deal of collateral damage. In other words, civilian casualties were sustainable and widespread. These indiscriminate bombings led Western aid organizations, the Western Alliance, and the rebel factions to accuse Russia of committing war crimes against the Syrian civilian population. These strikes also caused the displacement of tens of thousands of families from their homes. The flow of refugees grew, misery, and in destinations as the surrounding nations and aid organizations struggled to absorb the mass of humanity.

In April 2018, the Assad regime was yet again accused of new chemical attacks on the rebel-held northern town of Khan Sheikhoun where at least 80 people perished from the deadly gas. This was followed by another attack in the Eastern Ghouta town of Douma in April 2018 which killed another 40 people. The latter prompted the US, UK, and France to launch air strikes against chemical weapons facilities in Syria. Again, the regime denied the use of chemical weapons in their fight against rebel groups and was supported in Russia in their claimed innocence.

Meanwhile, in October 2017, Islamist militants lost control of the Syrian city of Raqqa, and in December 2018 the US government declared that Islamic State militants were defeated in Syria. This announcement was used by the US government as a justification for the US government's decision to pull out US troops from Syria. However, news reports claim that ISIS militants continue to control a small swath of land near the Euphrates River with a force of approximately 30,000 fighters (CNN, 2018).

This brief history of Syria, its authoritarian regime, and how its government has used lethal means to subvert democracy is a clear tale of the detrimental effects of authoritarian regimes, tribal, and exclusionary politics. Are Islamic State militants gone for good? Currently that is not a likely outcome. Insurgency is more likely given the Assad's regime heavy handed ways used to subvert democracy and quell any opposition. Today, Arab nations are making overtures to reconcile with Assad and readmit him to the fold of the Arab League, *a lesson not learned*. Russia continues is strong support for Assad and right-wing parties across Europe are also on friendly terms with Assad. These European parties see him as last defense against Islamist extremism. It seems like Syria is right back where it started eight years ago. The only difference is there are over a half a million dead, numerous cities in ruin, and half the population displaced. Authoritarian, tribal, and exclusionary rule remains.

5.5 Iraq

One can argue that Saddam Hussein's authoritarian rule has contributed significantly to the rise of Islamist jihadist terrorism and the establishment of the Islamic State in Iraq and Syria (ISIS) (Amonson, 2019). Saddam Hussein was president of Iraq from 1979 to 2003. He has been characterized as "the madman of the Middle East." He was barbaric and violent in treating his opposition, dangerous to the extreme. He ruled with an iron fist to maintain cohesion in a country with diverse ethnic groups and a long history of sectarian violence. He joined the Arab Baath Socialist Party in his early twenties and was engaged in assassination attempts on key Iraqi leaders opposing the Baath party. He was forced to flee to Egypt where he studied law and managed to rise in the ranks of the Egyptian Baath Party. He returned home in 1963 when the Baath Party gained power in Iraq.

In 1968 Sadaam Hussein became leader of the party and helped orchestrated a successful coup which made the Baath Party the political power house exerting political influence for 35 years. In 1979, Saddam Hussein became president. His regime was highly authoritarian. He ruled with violence and brutally exterminated opposition groups. An example of his ruthlessness is when his Minister of Health suggested that he may have to step down as president to reduce tension and conflict with Iran paving way for a peace treaty. Saddam arrested the minister and sent him home dismembered in a body bag the next day (Post, 2010, p. 343).

Although Sunnis served in his government, Kurds, Shias, and Christians were equally involved. However, religious activities were barely tolerated. He did not allow Sunni or Shia Islamist's teaching in schools. Arab nationalism, not Islamism, was the hallmark of Saddam's regime. Saddam's fall from power began when he invaded Kuwait in 1990 prompting a response from coalition forces led by the US. Saddam's forces were ejected from of Kuwait, but coalition forces consoled by then President George H. W. Bush allowed Saddam to remain in power. After the 2001 9/11 attacks in the US, the younger George W. Bush administration harbored a fear that that the next attack might be sourced from Iraq and Islamist terrorists may use weapons of mass destruction. Also, there were reports of a brutal repression of the Kurdish minority in northern Iraq. These reports included information that Saddam's forces had killed over 50,000 Kurds and destroyed thousands of Kurdish villages. In 2003, as a combination post 9/11 fear and intelligence used by the United States, an attack was launched in 2003 with the intent to topple Sadaam Hussein's regime. Saddam was captured and convicted by the Iraqi Special Tribunal and executed in December 2006.

In the subsequent months and years, the country then seemed to unravel. What had been a country built around national secular institutions, a sectarian war ensued. The war took on a variety of forms, but often built around the three factions of Sunnis, Shias, and Kurds. The U.S. occupation made attempts to establish a civil service structure to no avail. Civil authority broke down. U.S. troops left Iraq in 2011. The rise of the Islamic State ISIS followed. As Amonson (2019) puts it, after U.S. forces left Iraq in 2011, the country experienced seven years of intrastate conflict. The government was weak, security conditions were poor, economic development was stalled, sectarian violence increased, coupled with a large disenfranchised youth majority. These conditions flamed the fire of jihadist militancy.

By 2014 the Islamic State was established in territories of northern Iraq and Syria. Islamic State militants to practice their extremist religious beliefs and enforced a brutal version *sharia* law. Islamic State militants were able to seize vast swaths of territory and managed to establish a government structure with financial holdings comparable to a small country.

Today, the Islamic State is demolished. Iraq and coalition forces managed to retake much of the territory seized by Islamic State militants. However, there are signs that Islamic State militants are regrouping. Their attacks against government targets have increased from 2017 to 2018. The drivers that have created fertile ground for the rise of Islamists and Islamist militants have yet to be addressed, namely authoritarian, tribal, and exclusionary rule (Markusen, 2019).

5.6   Saudi Arabia

Saudi Arabia's authoritarian regime is blamed for many things, including Islamist extremism and militancy (Shane, 2016). The Saudi regime has long provided support for radical madrasa schools and mosques around the world that played a significant role in recruiting young people to join the Islamist jihad. These Saudi influences have managed to destroy tolerant Islamic traditions in several countries around the world. In news accounts from around the world the strict and narrow teaching in the madrasa schools around the world have been suspected of contributing to an Islamist view of the world. As part of that teaching and indoctrination of young men, the Saudis have been often blamed for facilitating the rise in Islamist jihadist violence. These Saudi supported schools and mosques preach an ultraconservative view of Islam: Wahhabism. This sect of Islam is a literalist, ultraconservative form of Sunni Islam. Adherents of Wahhabism often denigrate other the beliefs of other Islamic sects as well as the beliefs of Christians and Jews. Wahhabism is a rigid, patriarchal, and fundamentalist strain of Islam that many feels has fueled Islamist extremism and, in turn, an acceptance of Islamist jihadi terrorism. In countries like Pakistan and Nigeria, Saudi influence certainly seems to have translated into Islamist jihad terrorism. Wahhabism serves to dehumanize people of other faith as the word of God, hence making young Muslims more susceptible for recruitment by Islamist militants. Osama bin Laden and 15 of the 19 hijackers of 9/11 were Saudi citizens. Most of the suicide bombers who carried out terrorist operations in Iraq after the 2003 invasion were Saudi citizens. Saudi Arabia and Tunisia provided more foreign fighters to ISIS than any other country.

One can trace the history of the Wahhabi doctrine to 1964 when King Faisal took over the Saudi throne. Faisal, himself, was a modern man with Western views. He urged close ties with the West but failed to actively recognize the perils of the Wahhabi world view and act to reign in the Wahhabi influence. Over the next several decades, the Saudis financed the building of a great number of mosques and Islamic centers around the world spreading Wahhabism worldwide. Over the years, the Wahhabi's teachings became more puritanical, exclusionary, and dysfunctional (Wikipedia, 2019).

The year of the Islamic revolution in Iran, 1979, brought a powerful government and its goal of spreading Shia version of Islam. This was a major challenge to Saudi Arabia, the epicenter of the Sunni version of Islam. Saudi Arabia countered Iran's influence around the region and the world by investing in further promulgating Wahhabism around the world, and inadvertently exacerbating the radical Islamist jihadist movement. World events again provided an impetus to increased radicalization and Islamist political rise. In December 1979 the Soviet Union invaded Afghanistan to prop up the communist government. The resistance to the invasion came mostly from a band of local and MENA fighters, the mujahedeen, the warriors of Islam. To counter the Soviet occupation of Afghanistan the Saudi regime, with help from the US, was forced to provide logistical and lethal modern weapon support to the mujahedeen. A move that, inadvertently reinforced the battle cry of the Islamist jihadists. There was a war to be fought in the name of Islam. These mujahedeen are now the Taliban, the Islamist militants who to this very day are waging war in Afghanistan.

At the same time the Saudi regime treats Islamist jihadist terrorism as a menace as well as a direct threat to their Kingdom. They have joined Western regimes to denounce and act against Islamist jihadists and their violence (Shane, 2016). One senior Islamic cleric in Turkey reported that while he was meeting with Saudi clerics he became alerted to the fact that Saudi authorities had executed 47 people on terrorism charges in a single day, most of them were Saudi citizens. Since 2003, the regime has also acted more aggressively to clamp down on clerics who preach violent Islamist jihad. Cooperating with Western allies, they managed to curtail the supply of money to Islamic militants and foil terrorist plots. Thousands of imams were fired between 2004 and 2012 from their clerical posts for not doing enough to renounce extremism and curtail extremism from their rhetoric. Others (approximately 20,000) were ordered to participate in retraining programs.

Nevertheless, Saudi reform has moved excruciatingly slow. A study conducted by the International Center for Religion and Diplomacy completed a study in 2013 that reports the following:

> Seventh graders were being taught that "fighting the infidels to elevate the words of Allah" was among the deeds Allah loved the most, the report found, among dozens of passages it found troubling. Tenth graders learned that Muslims who abandoned Islam should be jailed for three days and, if they did not change their minds, "killed for walking away from their true religion." Fourth graders read that non-Muslims had been "shown the truth but abandoned it, like the Jews," or had replaced truth with "ignorance and delusion, like the Christians". (Shane, 2016)

Revisiting the authoritarian/tribal/exclusionary rule in Saudi Arabia and its role in propagating Islamist terrorism, we know that opposition to the Saudi royal family is not tolerated in any form. Islamist activists have been the most prominent threat to the regime. There are many terrorist incidents in Saudi Arabia that are not highly publicized (https://en.wikipedia.org/wiki/List_of_terrorist_incidents_in_Saudi_Arabia). Even peaceful protests are not allowed (https://en.wikipedia.org/wiki/Politics_of_Saudi_Arabia). More recently, crown prince Mohammed bin Salman, a royal member who is viewed as most powerful in the regime, was accused of funding extremism in the UK, violating human rights domestically, and causing famine for millions of people in Yemen as he wages war against the Shia Houthi population (Wintour & Davies, 2018). Furthermore, Salman has been accused of being complicit in the killing of Jamal Khashoggi, a critic of the royal regime and a columnist for the Washington Post (Aljazeera, 2019). Furthermore, recent news highlighted allegations that Saudi Arabia is heinously torturing female activists.[3] The activists seem to be advocating basic civil rights, such as women's right to drive. Allegations were made against the Saudi government namely that several activists were held in solitary confinement, they subjected to beatings, electric shocks, waterboarding, and sexual harassment.

5.7 Sudan

The final country examined in this look at MENA authoritarian regimes is Sudan. While not officially part of the MENA classification in many circles (For example, Sudan is classified as Sub-Saharan Africa by Freedom House and others). It is included here due its embracing Islamist groups and offering staging and safe-haven environments for a variety of groups. The government of Sudan is authoritarian and violently kleptocratic (Baldo, 2017). It is led by President Omar al-Bashir. Sudan's regime has a long history of religious persecution that continues today. Historically, the regime has provided tacit support to Islamist militant groups such as Hamas and al-Qaeda. Currently, the regime allows radical Islamist groups (al-Qaeda, Islamic State, Boko Haram, al-Shabab, etc.) to operate freely in Sudan. The regime runs a militia state and persecutes religious groups which do not subscribe to the regime's brand of Islam, namely Salafism (US Department of State, 2017a). The Salafist jihadi extremist groups operate freely all over Sudan under a complacent government. These groups have openly declared their support to ISIS. Most recently, *Time* magazine reported that Sudan is now experiencing an uprising that threatens to dismantle three decades of authoritarian rule (Baker, 2019). The authoritarian regime of Omar al-Bashir responded through a harsh crackdown on the protestors. A BBC documentary[4] provided detailed footage of protesters in Sudan being beaten and dragged away to secret detention facilities. These hit squads operate under the jurisdiction of the government secret services. The footage also describes the inhuman beatings and torture that occurs in these detention facilities.

The U.S. Commission on International Religious Freedom has designated Sudan as a "Country of Particular Concern" since 1999 (US Department of State, 2017b). Open Doors, a nonprofit organization which supports persecuted Christians around the globe, ranked Sudan the fifth worst country in the world for "extreme Christian persecution" in the 2017 World Watch list (Open Doors, 2017). International human rights organizations, such as Amnesty International and Human Rights Watch, have

---

[3]Post' View (2019). Saudi Arabia is heinously torturing female activists. It must face consequences. *The Washington Post* (retrieved from https://www.washingtonpost.com/opinions/global-opinions/saudi-arabia-is-heinously-torturing-female-activists-it-must-face-consequences/2019/02/10/67ac3e06-2b00-11e9-b2fc-721718903bfc_story.html?utm_term=.497cced75af0 on February 11, 2019).

[4]https://www.bbc.com/news/av/world-africa-47216487/what-happens-inside-sudan-s-secret-detention-centres.

amply documented attacks against the Christian minority in the country (see references in Baldo, 2017).

Most people in South Sudan are Christian and Animist. They struggled for decades against rule by the authoritarian rule of Omar al-Bashir and his Arab Muslim intolerant agenda. As a result, Sudan has been besieged by war and conflict. More than 1.5 million people perished because of this. Finally, people of the south of Sudan voted for independence in July 2011 creating two countries, namely Sudan (north) and South Sudan (BBC News, 2019).

5.8 Conclusion

A fundamental requirement for any effort by the offending party to create bridges and mend fences with the aggrieved party. Given that there may be a link between authoritarian/tribal/exclusionary regimes and the rise of Islamist jihadist terrorism, we believe that there must be a balance between the extent to which a government acts authoritatively to address Islamist grievances and at the same time combat Islamist terrorism. How can we envision this balance? Perhaps we can learn something from Tunisia.

Tunisia is the spark of the Arab Spring (the 2011 Arab uprisings against authoritarian rule, sometimes referred to as the "Jasmine Revolution"). Tunisia is also considered to have had a smoother transition from authoritarian rule to a form of democracy than other Arab countries such as Syria, Egypt, and Libya (Nada, 2017). After the Jasmine Revolution, Tunisia was able to institute democratic rule; although getting there was not easy. At first, there was conflict between secular and Islamist groups. The Islamist groups were mostly represented by the Ennahda (Renaissance) Party. The party brought together Islamist groups reflecting a wide spectrum—from Muslim democrats to Salafi ideologues to jihadi extremists (as in al-Qaeda and ISIS affiliates). Ennahda managed to obtain forty percent of the seats in parliament in the first post-revolutionary election in 2011. To accomplish this feat the party formed a coalition government with two secular parties. In 2013 Tunisia experienced a political crisis as the result of a political assassination of a leader of an opposition party. New elections took place in 2014 resulting in Ennahda winning a third of the seats in parliament.

In 2013, the economy sputtered, and Tunisians blamed Ennahda for the economic decline. In 2015, Tunisia was in a state of emergency. Jihadi terrorists struck in the heart of Tunisia—two secular politicians were assassinated by jihadi militants. Again, Ennahda was blamed for this atrocity. In 2014, Ennahda and another secularist party (Nidaa Tounes) formed a coalition government. The unity government has worked hard on economic reforms to boost the economy applying austerity measures. These measures proved unpopular by labor unions and opposition parties creating a wave of public negative sentiment toward the unity government. In 2016, the leadership of Ennahda made a strategic decision, namely to distance the party from the likes of al-Qaeda and ISIS. *They asserted that the party is about being a Muslim democrat.*

The renewed party recruited youth to its leadership ranks, adopted gender-parity legislation, and worked hard to coalesce with other governing parties to address the nation's economic problems. Additionally, the party allowed the passage of an anti-terrorism bill into law. Among the law provisions are:

- death penalty for convictions on terrorism charges,
- granting security forces broad powers to include monitoring and surveillance of suspected terrorist,
- extending incommunicado detention for terrorism suspects, and
- permitting courts to hold close hearings in cases related to terrorism charges (Nada, 2017).

Furthermore, the party cooperated with security forces to fight Tunisian Islamist jihadists trained in Libya, to dismantle countless Islamist jihadi cells, to crack down on imams deemed extremists, and to arrest thousands of Islamist terrorism suspects. The party also worked closely with the government to prevent radicalization through counter-messaging and educational programs.

Tunisia will forever go down in history as the birthplace of the Arab Spring in 2011. Tunisia has provided the world an experiment in using democratic means to combat radical Islamist jihadist terrorism. Could the same approach be adopted by other authoritarian/tribal/exclusionary regimes in the MENA region in culturally sensitive manners to the nations who populate the region and succeed? That is not to say that the Tunisia experiment in democracy and combatting jihadist terrorism is a total success. It is not by any means. Progress in Tunisia's democracy is slow, and some argue that progress has halted, perhaps due to the lack of economic progress. The unemployment rate for graduates is about 30%, wages are stagnant, and GDP per capita has declined since 2014 (Bremmer, 2019). Nevertheless, we can all learn from the Tunisia experiment. We learn that democracy works, but democracy by itself is not the panacea. Democracy interacts with a host of other institutional and societal factors in impact the quality of life of a country's citizenry. As such, democracy is foundational to combatting jihadist terrorism. Implicit in democracy is the protection of human rights (Parker, 2019). Governments react instinctively to the jihadist terrorism by reaching for the most coercive tools in their arsenal. This overreaction risks exacerbating the situation. This overreaction is driven by a lack of understanding of the true causes of jihadist terrorism. It is also driven by an erroneous assumption that the use of force will eradicate jihadist terrorism. Governments facing jihadist terrorism should put more faith in democracy and refraining from overreacting to the jihadist threat. A comprehensive and effective counterterrorism strategy should be grounded in respect for human rights and the rule of law.

References

al-Dali, F. (2011). Ḥiwār maᶜ al-Shaykh Sālim al-Shaykhi. *Ṣaḥifat ʾĀfāq, 1*(1), 6–7.

Aljazeera. (2019). Jamal Khashoggi case: All the latest updates. *Aljazeera*. Retrieved from https://www.aljazeera.com/news/2018/10/jamal-khashoggi-case-latest-updates-181010133542286.html on January 14, 2019.

Amonson, K. (2019). Iraq's power vacuum: A counterfactual analysis of Saddam Hussein's authoritarian rule. *Small Wars Journal*. Retrieved from https://smallwarsjournal.com/jrnl/art/iraqs-power-vacuum-counterfactual-analysis-saddam-husseins-authoritarian-rule on January 14, 2019.

Baker, A. (2019, February 4–11). An uprising in Sudan threatens to dismantle three decades of authoritarian rule. *Time*, p. 9.

Baldo, S. (2017). *Radical intolerance: Sudan's religious oppression and embrace of extremist groups*. The Enough Project. Retrieved from https://enoughproject.org/wp-content/uploads/2017/12/SudanReligiousFreedom_Enough_Dec2017_final.pdf on January 14, 2019.

Bellin, E. (2004). The robustness of authoritarianism in the Middle East. *Comparative Politics, 36*(2), 139–157.

Bellin, E. (2012). Authoritarianism in the Middle East: Lessons from the Arab Spring. *Comparative Politics, 44*(2), 127–149.

BBC News. (2019). Sudan country profile. *BBC News*. Retrieved from https://www.bbc.com/news/world-africa-14094995 on January 15, 2019.

Boduszyński, M. P. (2015). The external dimension of Libya's troubled transition: The international community and 'democratic knowledge' transfer. *Journal of North African Studies, 20*(5), 735–753.

Boix, C. (2011). Democracy, development, and the international system. *American Political Science Review, 105*(4), 809–828.

Bremmer, I. (2019, February 4–11). Tunisia's fledgling democracy shows signs of wear and tear. *Time*, p. 19.

CNN. (2018). ISIS fast facts. *CNN Library*, December 20, 2018. Retrieved from https://www.cnn.com/2014/08/08/world/isis-fast-facts/index.html on January 13, 2019.

Crenshaw, M. (2011). *Explaining terrorism: Causes, processes and consequences*. New York: Routledge.

Dalacoura, K. (2012). The 2011 uprisings in the Arab Middle East: Political change and geopolitical implications. *International Affairs, 88*(1), 63–79.

Encyclopedia Britannica. (2018). Syrian civil war. *Encyclopedia Britannica*. Retrieved from https://www.britannica.com/event/Syrian-Civil-War on January 13, 2019.

Goldberg, E. (2018, August 15). Egypt's new political system of one: Its president. *The Washington Post*. https://www.washingtonpost.com/news/monkey-cage/wp/2018/08/15/egypts-new-political-system-of-one-its-president/?noredirect=on&utm_term=.0f18235050d5.

Kamrava, M. (2013). From Territories to Independent States. In *The modern Middle East: A political history since the First World War* (pp. 35–67). University of California Press.

Markusen, M. B. (2019). The Islamic State and the persistent threat of extremism in Iraq. *CSIS Briefs*. Retrieved from https://www.csis.org/analysis/islamic-state-and-persistent-threat-extremism-iraq on January 14, 2019.

Martin, G. (2018). *Understanding terrorism: Challenges, perspectives, and issues* (6th ed.). Los Angeles: Sage Publications.

Nada, G. (2017). The Islamist spectrum—Tunisia: From democrats to jihadist. Wilson Center. Retrieved from https://www.wilsoncenter.org/article/the-islamist-spectrum-tunisia-democrats-to-jihadis on January 15, 2019.

Obeidi, A. S. (2008). *al-Thaqāfah al-Siyāsiyah fi Libyā [Political culture in Libya]*, Trans. M. Z. al-Mghayrbi. Benghazi: University of Garyounis.

Open Doors. (2017). *World Watch List*. Available at https://www.opendoorsusa.org/christian-persecution/worldwatch-list/. Last accessed November 2017.

Pargeter, A. (2009). Localism and radicalization in North Africa: Local factors and the development of political Islam in Morocco, Tunisia and Libya. *International Affairs, 85*(5), 1031–1044.

Parker, T. (2019). *Avoiding the terrorist trap: Why respect for human rights is the key to defeating terrorism.* New Jersey: World Scientific/WorldSciNet.

Pillar, P. R. (2001). *Terrorism and U.S. foreign policy.* Washington, DC: Brooking Institution Press.

Post, J. (Ed.). (2010). *The psychological assessment of political leaders: With profiles of Saddam Hussein and Bill Clinton.* An Arbor: University of Michigan Press.

Sawani, Y. M. (2012). Post-Qadhafi Libya: Interactive dynamics and the political future. *Contemporary Arab Affairs, 5*(1), 1–26.

Shane, S. (2016). Saudis and extremism: Both the arsonists and the firefighters. *The New York Times.* Retrieved from https://www.nytimes.com/2016/08/26/world/middleeast/saudi-arabia-islam.html on January 14, 2019.

Shehata, D. (2009). *Islamists and secularists in Egypt: Opposition, conflict and cooperation.* London: Routledge.

Stansfield, G. (2013). The unravelling of the post-First World War state system? The Kurdistan Region of Iraq and the transformation of the Middle East. *International Affairs, 89*(2), 259–282.

The American Foreign Policy Council's World Almanac of Islamism. (2018). *Libya.* Retrieved from http://almanac.afpc.org/Libya on January 13, 2019.

Toaldo, M. (2016). Decentralizing authoritarianism? The international intervention, the new 'revolutionaries' and the involution of Post-Qadhafi Libya. *Small Wars & Insurgencies, 27*(1), 39–58.

U.S. Department of State. (2017a). *Sudan 2016 international religious freedom report.* Available at https://www.state.gov/documents/organization/268944.pdf.

U.S. Department of State. (2017b). *Frequently asked questions: IRF report and countries of particular concern.* Available at https://www.state.gov/j/drl/irf/c13003.htm. Last accessed September 2017.

Walsh, D. (2019, February 14). Egypt's parliament clears way for El-Sisi to rule until 2034. *The New York Times.* Retrieved from https://www.nytimes.com/2019/02/14/world/middleeast/egypt-sisi.html on February 14, 2019.

Wikipedia. (2019). Politics of Saudi Arabia. *Wikipedia.* Retrieved from https://en.wikipedia.org/wiki/Politics_of_Saudi_Arabia on January 14, 2019.

Wintour, P., & Davies, C. (2018). Saudi crown prince's UK visit prompts heavy criticism by opposition. *The Guardian.* Retrieved from https://www.theguardian.com/uk-news/2018/mar/07/saudi-crown-prince-uk-visit on January 14, 2019.

Yom, S. L. (2016). *From resilience to revolution: How foreign interventions destabilize the Middle East.* New York: Columbia University Press.

Chapter 6
Globalization, the Media, and Islamist Jihad

Abstract This chapter discusses five major themes in this chapter directly related to globalization, the media, and their effects on the rise jihadist terrorism in the last 4–5 decades. These themes are (1) globalization and the breakdown of the welfare state; (2) globalization, consumerism, and postmodernism; (3) negative media portrayals of Islam and Muslims in Western and global media, (4) the use of global media by Wahhabis and Jihadi terrorists; and (5) the effects of media owned and operated by political Islamists.

Keywords Globalization · Global media · Welfare state · Consumerism · Postmodernism · Wahhabism · Media portrayals of Muslims · Jihadist terrorism

6.1 Introduction

> The coverage of Islam in the media is becoming more sophisticated, and there is more access to knowledge.
>
> Leila Aboulela[1]

In Chap. 1 we argued that globalization can bring about marginalization of members of societies when their countries fail in delivering a standard of living equal to the global norm, in which the norm is clearly articulated and publicized through the various global media. Marginalized people become acutely aware of their backwardness by witnessing the standard of living (and potentially the perceived decadence and political indifference) of people in the developed world. In this chapter, we explore the notion that globalization and global media could be drivers in the rise of Islamist jihadist terrorism in the MENA region. Specifically, we will discuss five interrelated themes of globalization and global media. These are (1) globalization and the breakdown of the welfare state; (2) globalization, consumerism, and postmodernism; (3) negative media portrayals of Islam and Muslims in Western and global media; (4) the use of global media by Wahhabis and Jihadi terrorists; and (5) the effects of media owned and operated by political Islamists.

---

[1] https://www.brainyquote.com/quotes/leila_aboulela_730243.

© Springer Nature Switzerland AG 2019   113
M. J. Sirgy et al., *Combatting Jihadist Terrorism through Nation-Building*, Human Well-Being Research and Policy Making, https://doi.org/10.1007/978-3-030-17868-0_6

6.2 Globalization and the Breakdown of the Welfare State

One can argue that the catalyst of the Iranian revolution in the early 1980s and the rise of Islamist movements was a "war against modernity" (Lewis, 1990). In such a way of thinking, the Iranian revolution and the rise of Islamist movements throughout the MENA region and beyond was, in part, driven by disaffection of various MENA populations feeling ostracized by their governments and outside influencers who were disregarding "core moral and religious aspects" of Islam in their push toward rapid modernization. The basic tenet underlying the evolution of the Islamic Republic of Iran and the Islamist movements that followed is the rejection of modern life and the return to the early perceived glorious days of medieval Islam (Ahmed, 1992; Ahmed & Donnan, 1994; Ayubi, 1991; Esposito, 1992; Gellner, 1992; Roy, 1994; Turner, 1994; Voll, 1994; Zubaida, 1993).

The era of "postmodernity" as some scholars call it, is seen as the abandonment of the welfare state, the development of Keynesian welfare, globalization of government deregulation, and the reinstatement of economic neo-liberalism. One can argue that a key factor related to the rise of Islamist movements is the breakdown and abandonment of the welfare state in the MENA region. World-wide we started witnessing postmodernism in the mid-1970s. Post modernity is often seen as a social condition of late capitalism (Turner, 1994). The most prominent characteristic of postmodernity is the decline of social Keynesianism, defined as "disorganized capitalism" (Lash & Urry, 1987; Offe, 1985) or "risk society" (Beck, 1992). In such an era, there is a witnessing of a decline of welfare capitalism, increased political attacks on the legitimacy of social security, and the globalization of government deregulation. During that period, "uncertainties of deregulated economy have produced incalculable levels of risk for modern individuals" (Turner, 1994, p. 182). One can argue that disorganized capitalism was a function of the same precursors that led to the fall of the Soviet Union in 1991. A revolutionary wave in the late 1980s and early 1990s ended communist rule in Central and Eastern Europe and beyond. The breakdown of the Soviet system signaled the end of communism and the triumph of capitalism. The disintegration of the Soviet Union and the collapse of the state socialist system reinforced the Western models of development as key to modernization world-wide. Unfortunately, the capitalism that gripped many countries, including those that made up the Soviet empire and China at that time was indeed chaotic (Lane, 1999; Shlapentokh, 2017). Living standards declined markedly in those countries making the transition from communism to capitalism. Consulting firms, global funding institutions like the International Monetary Fund (IMF), and Western banks demanded economic solutions be imposed on these former and current communist regimes without recognizing the societal earthquakes they were unleashing in these societies. The welfare system that provided economic security to the masses was all but gone in the name of economic reform and the need for austerity. The emergence of Islamist movements seems to be a direct result of the chaos of this period—a period characterized by historians and political scientists as "disorganized capitalism" and "risk society."

Consider what happened in Egypt in the mid-1970s. President Anwar El-Sadat and the IMF instituted the Open-Door Economic policy, the *Infitah*, in the mid-1970s (Abdel-Khalek, 1981; Baker, 1981; Dessouki, 1981). This policy amounted to an attack on the Keynesian welfare state by abandoning goods and currency subsidies. The Islamist movement in Egypt became increasingly popular in the way the movement dealt with the adverse repercussion of the *Infitah* doctrine by providing social services (such as clinics, schools and banks) to people whose livelihood was threatened by the new postmodernism. That is, Islamist groups stepped into the social breach torn open in the name of economic reform and provided much needed social program security when security was compromised in the newly established modern society.

The Islamist movements' replacement of long-standing social safety nets and care for the lower classes in society with their own institutions gave them a great deal of social power in the eyes of the middle and lower classes. The rise of the Islamic State (ISIS) in Syria and Iraq was successful, in part, because of these Islamist social institutions (Al-Tamimi, 2014). ISIS managed to build and run schools, a court system, law enforcement, and provide services to the poor (e.g., distribution of bread free of charge). The political strategy of offering expected social capital that had been swept aside by Western and existing governments through reborn social services is considered the model for current and future Islamist jihadists seeking to occupy territory in a lawless environment where government forces relinquished control.

An examination of the timeline of development of Islamist social institutions seems to indicate that this is a key in the spread of the Islamist doctrine among the middle and lower classes in the MENA region (Clark, 2004). Examples of Islamic social institutions in the region include Islamic medical clinics in Cairo, the Women's Committee of the Islah Charitable Society in Yemen, and the Islamic Center Charitable Society in Jordan. These institutions played an important role in the recruitment of the poor, as well as the middle class, into the Islamist jihadist ranks. They did this by creating associating their good deeds with Islamist extremism.

6.3 Globalization, Consumerism, and Postmodernism

It can be argued that another key factor related to the rise of Islamist movements is *globalization* itself. A significant element of globalization is the increased diffusion of new technologies of mass communication that connected the most remote parts of the world through information (Ahmed & Donnan, 1994). Capitalist goods and services have been made more accessible than ever before and information about the consumption of these goods and services became increasingly omnipresent. That is, information and images of hedonistic consumption became pervasive and ubiquitous through of plethora of media sources. Such relentless information and images of postmodern consumption created a major negative externality, namely the impression that the West has now a large imprint on the cultural and political landscape of global society through an ever-increasing consumerism. Reacting to this worldwide consumerism, Islamists feared that participation in this consumer culture would lead to the disintegration of Muslim culture and the fragmentation of Muslim beliefs and values. "Consumerism offers or promises a range of possible lifestyles which compete with, and in many respects, contradict the uniform lifestyle demanded by Islamic fundamentalism" (Turner, 1994, p. 90). The image of the "good life" as widely disseminated through global media puts the "mosque" and the "mall" at odds. "In the present modernist era, the mall for the Americans is the contemporary equivalent of the mosque. It acts as a social focus, and people go to it faithfully, daily, for renewal and companionship" (Ahmed, 1992, p. 208). Islamic clerics and religious leaders treated the images of the bourgeois way of life focusing on leisure, gratification, and hedonism transmitted through global media as a major threat to an Islamic way of life. One that is centered on a religious core. While not necessarily an austere life, it could be certainly considered a reflective and spiritually focused one.

A distinction must be made between Islam and Islamism. Traditional Islam prescribes rules of individual behavior that would help pave way to salvation in the afterlife. In contrast, Islamism seeks a new world order, a political economy guided by Islamic principles (Pipes, 2002). Islamism can be described in terms of three pillars: (1) a devotion to Islamic principles as revealed by the *Qur'an*, (2) a rejection of Western culture, and (3) the transformation of Islamic principles into an ideology and political economy. Islamists reject many aspects of Western influence: Western philosophy, Western customs and values, and Western institutions of all types —political, economic, social, technological, educational, and cultural are all subject to an intense examination and reinterpretation that links them to an Islamist doctrine. Islamists will often preach virulent mistrust and rejection of the West because of the West's domineering influence in all aspects of the global modern life. In addition, they may well hold onto an historical rivalry with the West in the rise and nurturing of all human civilization.

6.4 Negative Media Portrayals of Islam and Muslims in Western and Global Media

The global media also played a major role in communicating to the Muslim public worldwide how Muslim immigrants and refugees are treated in Western countries. Not a flattering image; an image that breeds Muslim anger and resentment toward Westerners (El-Aswad, 2013).

During the last three decades we have witnessed negative portrayals of Islam and Muslims by Western media, media organizations that have turned into global media—the media that Muslim publics around the world are exposed to (Poole & Richardson, 2006; Saeed, 2007; Zelizer & Allan, 2002). The images and representations of Islam and Muslims in mainstream Western media have been mostly demeaning and hostile. For example, Muslims in Britain are frequently characterized as "un-British" (Saeed, 2004). In certain circles (and media) Muslims have consistently been identified and labeled as outsiders whose culture is alien and incompatible with the British culture. Some see British culture as one that could describe as "Christian and white." Similar findings highlighting the negative views of Islam and Muslims held by certain groups and media show up in a variety of other Western countries such as Canada (El-Masry, 2002), Australia (Manning 2006), the European Union (Fekete, 2002). Allen and Nielsen (2002, p. 47) summarized the research in the European Union as follows: "The media's role cannot be overlooked, and it has been identified as having an inherent negativity towards Muslims and Islam."

Books that are translated into many languages and widely disseminated are also part of the global media. In this context there are many books in the global media that characterize Muslims and Islam as a threat to Western civilization. A clear example is Samuel Huntington's book on *Clash of Civilizations*. Huntington (1997) has long argued that there is a cold war between Western and Muslim culture, and that Islam preaches violence and Muslims have an innate propensity to violence. Huntington's view is basically that, Muslims are inherently inferior. Sardar and Davies (2002) illustrate how Huntington's argument has been used in the global media:

> On December 3, 2001, issue of the National Review, with a drawing of George Bush as a medieval crusader on the cover contained an article headlined 'Martyred: Muslim Murder and Mayhem against Christians' in which the author cites with the approval the conclusion in Samuel Huntington's book, The Clash of Civilizations and the Remaking of World Order: "The underlying problem for the West is not Islamic fundamentalism. It is Islam, a different civilization whose people are convinced of the superiority of their culture and are obsessed with the inferiority of their power". (p. 49)

Muslims, and particularly Arab Muslims, are found to be near the bottom of many quality-of-life metrics (Pipes, 2002). They are rated poorly in terms of military prowess, political stability, economic development, human rights, health and longevity, education and literacy, corruption, among others. When such ratings are highly publicized in the global media, Muslims around the world, and particularly Arab Muslims, are presented with a feeling that the world views them as inferior and contributes to, whether true or not, a sense of cultural inferiority. These feelings are accentuated given the fact that Arab Muslims had once enjoyed what could clearly be rated as a superior civilization. One which led the world in a variety of areas including scientific study and mathematics. During this golden era dating back to the seventh and eighth centuries, Arab Muslims conquerors managed to assemble an empire extending from Spain in the west to India in the east. Arab Muslims built a vast and proud civilization which had borrowed the best from a wealth of lands they had brought under the Muslim banner. For many Arab Muslims, this history creates a bitter pill to swallow regarding a modern Islam culture in the MENA region. When compared to its history the modern Islam appears to be an unmistakable failure compared to medieval successes. This perception is one which has been leveraged in the narrative presented by the Islamist movement. It is also one which calls for a rebirth of this golden era through rejection of a modernity imposed by Western based ideals and an embracing of "the true path' through strict adherence to the ways of Islam as interpreted by ultra-conservative sects within Islam.

6.5   The Use of Global Media by Wahhabis and Islamist Jihadi Terrorists

Wahhabism is a brand of Islam which advocates that the world is divided between devout believers of worldwide community of Muslim brothers and sisters (*ummah*) and evil non-believers, viewed as infidels, apostates, and heretics.[2] Non-believers include all non-Muslims, including Jews, Christians, and fellow Muslims who do not subscribe to the literal interpretation of the Qur'an, as well as those whose beliefs, values, and lifestyle reflects Western customs and ideals.

Wahhabi clerics and religious leaders used a mix of global media as a countervailing force against Western consumerism and postmodernism. They forcefully used global media to implement the mission of Wahhabism, the eighteenth-century call to homogenize Islamic traditions into a single universal system worldwide. Schwartz (2005) contends that a great many of the mosques in America are funded through Saudi Wahabi sources. The sect also funds a great many programs and organizations that provide Islamic chaplains to the prison systems in the United States, and a variety of organizations (e.g. The Islamic Society of North America) that speak to United States media outlets in the name of Islam. The Wahabis also mobilized the Muslim *ummah* (the global community of Muslims) to defend the Islamic way of life.

Since the mid-1970s, the global media have been used to spread the Wahhabi brand of Islam by hammering at the message that Islam is a global culture and a global way of life that should replace Western consumerism and the Western way of life. Let us focus on one jihadist organization, namely Al-Qaeda. Ciovacco (2009) notes that Al-Qaeda has its own media wing, Al-Sahab. The purpose of Al-Sahab is to basically "connect" to the world. Combined with a few multiple media outlets such as the Global Islamic Media Front, Al-Qaeda has put together a media infrastructure to support its followers and inspire potential recruits. This infrastructure connects a diverse and widespread group of Islamists and provides a well-financed and skilled communication and propaganda network for furthering both the short-term and long-term goals of Al-Qaeda and related Islamist groups. As Ciovacco puts it,

> Al-Qaeda Central employs a cogent media strategy to communicate with its affiliates, win over mainstream Muslims, and inspire the "true believers" into action against the perceived enemies of Islam. Al-Qaeda has crafted this media strategy during a global marketing campaign against the United States. (p. 853)

We will spend the next part of this chapter examining how this organization used global media to spread Wahhabism world-wide. Al-Qaeda has been very successful in using global media, particularly the Internet, in spreading Wahhabism brand of Islam and recruit members in local terror cells all over the globe. The Al-Qaeda network used multiple formats such as Internet postings, audio recordings, video releases, and published articles in a global dissemination of their rhetoric (Fucito, 2006).

---

[2]See "Analysis Wahhabism" in *Saudi Time Bomb?* PBS Frontline, November, 2001. http://www.pbs.org/wgbh/pages/frontline/shows/saudi/.

Al-Qaeda's communication strategy involved multiple audiences throughout the Middle East, Europe, Asia, and the United States. Their message varies as a direct function of the issues of the time. They issued demands, made threats, and made warning announcements of specific terror action directed against political and ideological enemies such as governments of the United States, Saudi Arabia, Israel, and Iraq. Another audience is the average Arab Muslim in the MENA region, those reluctant to support jihadist actions. Messages directed to this audience typically involve Quranic justification of Islamist jihadist violence against the "enemies of Islam" as well as fear message. The following is an example of a fear message:

> … the U.S., in conjunction with its puppet states in the region and Israel, is waging a war against Islam, particularly through its policies in the Israeli-Palestinian conflict, its support for sanctions on Iraq and its military presence in the Gulf region. (Brown, 2003, p. 95)

Inducing fear by persuading their audience that Islam is in jeopardy and Muslims' lives are at stake can be highly persuasive. Exploiting Arab Muslim's attitude about the incessant Israeli-Palestinian conflict offers a cogent and appealing persuasive message. It can be focused on how the United States has long supported Israel, the enemy of all Muslims, and suppressed the inalienable rights of the Palestinians. As such, the United States government and its people must be deterred and pay the price for their malfeasance. The Palestinian cause is used as a catalyst to gain universal Arab support for the Islamist jihad against the United States. Islamist Jihadist terrorists want to frighten people. Fear motivates people to put pressure on institutions that might assuage their fears. For example, the Al-Qaeda network issues warnings detailing pending attacks against target populations and institutions. Again, these pronouncements are designed to induce fear, creating a sense of urgency to act to counteract the impending destruction. Yet another fear strategy is the release of gruesome video and still images of hostage beheadings and human carnage in the aftermath of a specific terrorist attack.

> Fear has changed the outcomes of recent European elections, impacted foreign policies, lead to the withdrawal of foreign troops in Iraq, and fractured international alliances. Fear has provided terrorist networks with a substantial source of hard power. (Nye, 2004, p. 14)

Still another important audience include wealthy Muslims who have the financial means to support the Islamist jihadist cause. There is yet another audience comprised of members of terror cells ("sleeper cells") who are ready and willing to carry out terrorist action against specific institutional targets throughout the world. What the numbers are is not clear, but speculation runs from a dozen or so to hundreds. The end of the Syrian civil war may well lead to an increase in these numbers as foreign fighters return to their own countries.

The selection of the specific terror targets in terms of place and time is also a key ingredient in the media strategy. Specifically, Al-Qaeda operatives would launch an attack in areas and at times most conducive to leverage global media—the news media covering the terror events. As such, this media strategy assures maximum publicity through global media. Besides the strategic use of news media in this horrific way, Al-Qaeda's media strategy relied heavily on the Internet. Al-Qaeda's operatives routinely hijacked network servers of unsuspecting institutions to post messages that are untraceable.

> Jihadis are using the Internet and the Web to inspire the creation of a virtual global tribe of Islamic radicals – an online *umma* with kinship segments around the world. (Ronfeldt, 2005, p. 18)

In the context of the Internet, Al-Qaeda is notorious for its use of social networking sites. Al-Qaeda terrorists have managed to set up sites such as Jihad Videos to spread their lethal ideology and provide links to additional websites. They were successful in creating "a virtual community of hatred" in cyberspace (Hunt, 2006). Operatives have managed to plan and carry out attacks using surreptitious e-mail servers (Coll & Glasser, 2005). Ironically, Al-Qaeda operatives have also used the Internet as a research tool by gathering information on target sites and institutions such as nuclear power plant layouts, railway maps, water supply networks, airport flight schedules—information available for the public on the Internet (McGeough, 2006a). Operatives have also managed to upload videos on the Internet to serve many terrorist goals. Al-Qaeda's complete *Encyclopedia of Jihad* can be downloaded from the Internet, for example (McGeough, 2006b).

It is obvious that Al-Qaeda ran a well scripted global media program. The target populations go beyond the geographic bounds of the MENA region. They reach across a great many varied landscapes and cultures. They have, however, shown that they do understand the marketing of their brand of Islam. They provide a consistent set of messages that can be used to reach to the core beliefs of their diverse global audiences. At the same time, they can adapt their messages to take advantage of geographical or demographic segments around the world. In that manner they seek to connect on a common core of faith but adjust the message around a local theme. A strategy that has served global consumer product companies well over the decades of globalization of markets. We continue our examination by looking at the use of media on a more regional and local basis. In these cases, more traditional media outlets and control of flow of information has been co-opted and exploited by several different Islamist entities.

6.6   The Effect of Media Owned and Operated by Political Islamists

A significant factor in the rise of Islamist extremism and jihadist terrorism is the promulgation of media owned and operated by political Islamists. We have seen this in many MENA countries. A case in point is Iraq (Al-Marashi, 2006/2007). The tension among ethnic Kurds, Turkmens and Arabs, and Sunni and Shi'a Muslim sects are fueled by the fact that local media are formed along ethno-sectarian lines. As such, the local media have reinforced the country's ethno-sectarian divisions.

As reported by Al-Marashi (2006/2007), during the Ba'ath era (i.e., Saddam Hussein's authoritarian regime), there were five state-owned newspapers and one television channel. In the post Saddam era, we witnessed the emergence of hundreds of newspapers and several satellite channels. These media outlets have exacerbated Iraq's ethno-sectarian conflict. Ethnic factions gained their own means of communicating to their ethno-sectarian constituencies in Iraq and abroad (the Iraqi diaspora). In particular, political Islamists owned and operated their own media (radio stations, newspapers, and satellite channels).

For example, the Al-Furat satellite channel, based in Baghdad, began broadcasting in November 2004. It is owned and operated by a prominent Shi'a Islamist political faction, namely the Supreme Council for the Islamic Revolution in Iraq (SCIRI). News reports and commentaries in Al-Furat have frequently referred to victimization by Sunni Arab militants (e.g., members of the Al-Qaeda organization in Iraq). Coverage of inter-sectarian violence against Iraqi Shi'a Muslims is pervasive in Al-Furat's programs. In contrast, the dominant frame of the Arab Sunni media (e.g., Rafidayn Channel and The Baghdad Satellite Channel) is "resistance" to "occupation forces" (i.e., the US military). Much of the rhetoric that stems from the Arab Sunni media reflects a "foreign scheme to divide the nation." Arab Sunni Muslims fear a land grab by the Kurds in the north and Shi'a Muslims in the south leaving the Arab Sunnis in a landlocked poor state. Furthermore, Arab Sunni media have consistently referred to insurgents as "armed men" rather than "terrorists." Arab Sunni media have also focused on the plight of Iraqi prisoners, many of them are Arab Sunnis and regarded as "political prisoners."

What could be considered one of the worst media outlets calling for violence is Al-Zawra. This outlet is a satellite channel that serves as a mouthpiece for the Iraqi politician, Mish'an al-Juburi. The outlet has essentially evolved into a platform for Islamist jihadist terrorism. The slogan of Mish'an al-Juburi is "The voice of the excluded and marginalized." The station regularly broadcasts footage of terrorists' attacks against multinational forces and the Iraqi government. The station makes announcements that incite violence by calling on Iraqis to join the "jihad" against the United States and Iran and their sympathizers. Most of the news footage is provided by Islamist jihadi militants such as the Islamic Army in Iraq. The government ordered the closure of the station on charges of inciting violence. However, the station was able to circumvent closure by using transnational satellites with many centers in Iraq protected by Islamist insurgents. Foreign reporters have designated Al-Zawra as an "Al-Qaeda channel" although its relationship with the Al-Qaeda organization in Iraq is tenuous at best (Howard, 2007). Most disturbingly, it was reported that a Saudi cleric has issued *fatwas* (religious mandates) calling for Saudis to watch "the channel of the Mujahidin" (religiously inspired fighters), asserting that, "it teaches the art of jihad, a matter the youth of our *Umma* [religious community] desperately need" (Open Source Center, 2007).

Given the importance of the media in inciting Islamist jihadist terrorism, Al-Marashi (2006/2007) made the following recommendations. First, the Iraqi media landscape should be assessed by creating a national media directory of all local media and conducting a media consumption assessment (the size and composition of the audience of each media outlet). Second, the previous action should be followed by improving and implementing media regulation. A prime example of media regulation is the ban on spreading sectarian, racial, and religious sedition and strife. The existing broadcasting code of practice (the code designed to encourage the reporting of ethno-sectarian issues) should be codified by government legislation and government administration of these regulations. International assistance should be encouraged by creating an Iraqi media loan fund as well as an Iraqi media development network. Third, there should be better media education. This is critical. Medi education should include improved through the implementation of a program of aimed at training for Iraqi media practitioners and improving local media educational institutions. Fourth, Iraqi journalists and their families need to be better protected by civil authorities and police forces. Finally, a "peace media" alternative should be created. This can be done by learning from other applied experiences in peace media. (For an example see Rawan & Hussain, 2017) Developing a peace media strategy, focusing attention on entertainment (rather than news about political issues and military operations), and translating literature on peace media into Arabic, Kurdish, and Turkish and distributing this literature at media institutions and educational facilities.

The MENA region and the United States are not alone in Islamist radicalization programs through a variety of traditional media, social media, and more traditional personal appeals through a variety of funded organizations. The global nature of these platforms provides a world- wide stage upon which to offer their extremist versions of what being a Muslim demand. They are active in all parts of the Muslim world. In Indonesia, the largest Muslim country in the world, Muljadji, Sekarningrum, and Muhammad (2017) report how manipulation of social media platforms have been used to support the strict interpretation of Islam and what that requires of individuals. They provide an example of how this has impacted daily lives in even such things as clothing and dress. They note one example of this regarding young women's views as wearing the hijab. The authors report an increase in social media active women viewing those who do not wear the hijab or veil as infidels. Bardos (2014) discusses the coordinated process and programs directed at Muslims in the Balkans of Europe. The author relates how one of the most moderate Muslim populations in the world has been targeted by Islamists since Yugoslavia broke apart in a vicious civil war. Social media platforms and well-funded and used effectively. Bardos (p. 46) notes:

> Militant Islamists in the Balkans have developed an extensive array and network of print periodicals, bookstores, websites, and YouTube spots spreading religious intolerance, glorifications of violence, and anti-American, anti-Semitic, anti-democratic messages. Islamic bookstores from Belgrade to Novi Pazar distribute tracts by extremists such as the contemporary Islamist ideologue Yusuf al-Qaradawi and the mid-century Marx of Islamism Sayyid Qutb. Militant Islamist websites promote jihad, suicide bombings, and the killing of non-Muslims. (p. 46)

The Islamist Jihadists who flocked to the Caliphate in Syria and Iraq are now potentially returning to their homelands around the world. Once returned to their homelands, they will have easy access to the messages and continued calls to Islamist Jihad through this complex and well-established global media presence. For example there were several fighters who went to Syria and Iraq from the Balkans. Quotes from some of these give local governments a great deal of concern regarding these radicalized fighters intentions once they return home to Europe and other parts of the world.

6.7   Summary and Conclusion

In this chapter we identified and briefly discussed five major themes related to globalization, the media, and their effects on the rise Islamist Jihadist terrorism: (1) globalization and the breakdown of the welfare state; (2) globalization, consumerism, and postmodernism; (3) negative media portrayals of Islam and Muslims in Western and global media, (4) the use of global media by Wahhabis and Islamist Jihadist terrorists; and (5) the effects of media owned and operated by political Islamists. With respect to the first theme, we argued that the world has witnessed the disintegration of a long standing welfare state in many countries of the MENA region. A disintegration that could be considered as a direct function of the fall of communism and the dismantling of the Soviet empire. This event left a gaping economic and social support hole for a significant portion of the population that was filled by social services provided by Islamist organizations. These social service institutions managed to win the hearts and minds of many moderate middle-class and poor Muslims and, in turn, helped to radicalize them. As such, we believe that the social services provided by organizations such as the Muslim Brotherhood have been an important catalyst and sustaining influence in the rise of Islamist Jihadist terrorism.

Regarding the impact of globalization, consumerism, and postmodernism, we believe these trends have also played an important role in the promulgation of Islamist movements. Globalization, consumerism, and postmodernism are equated in the sense that the postmodern era (1970s and beyond) was marked by a global society with rampant and crass consumerism. Consumers in the developed world enjoyed goods and services that the vast majority of people in the developing world felt were beyond all their means and hope. Images of rampant consumption were highly publicized through the global media making deprived Muslims resentful of this clear flouting of wealth and consumer culture. Muslim clerics revolted against this decadence from the West and advocated against hedonistic consumption. In lieu of consumerism, they advocated a political economy based on conservative Islamic principles, a global Islamist movement to replace the decadent Western system.

Negative portrayals of Islam and Muslims in western and global media can also be seen to have played a key role in the rise of Islamist Jihadist terrorism. Muslims were exposed to images and informed through the news media about prejudice and discrimination against their fellow Muslim brethren in their own countries and more importantly in the West. Muslim immigrants and refugees are mistreated in Western countries and the media were full of scenes of political leaders and others indicating that Muslims were not welcome. News videos displayed crowds and leaders making it clear that Muslims should go home to where they came from. Knowing about the mistreatment of their brethren created a great deal of Muslim anger and resentment toward Westerners.

The strategic use of global media by Wahhabis and Islamist Jihadi operatives contributed as well to the rise of Islamist terrorism and the support for it in the MENA region as well as globally. Wahhabism, as previously noted, is an ultra-conservative brand of Islam that can breed intolerance and hatred toward evil non-believers—infidels, apostates, and heretics to include all non-Muslims, Jews, Christians, and fellow Muslims who do not subscribe to the literal interpretation of the Qur'an, as well as those whose beliefs, values, and lifestyle reflect Western customs and ideals. Wahhabi clerics and religious leaders have been quite successful in their well-funded and strategic use of both local and global media, spreading this intolerant and potentially toxic version of Islam to a wide audience of Muslims around the world. Organizations such as Al-Qaeda were very successful in operating an effective global marketing campaign which used a variety of integrated elements that leveraged a mix of targeted messages of fear and hate to mobilize vulnerable Muslims against Western people, thought, and institutions. They had a well-constructed and managed multi-media presence that involved the vast social media platforms available on the internet to influence thought, recruit militants, secure funding, and plan and execute terrorist operations. Their effective use of the modern global media landscape is clearly an important factor in the rise of Islamist Jihadist terrorism.

The final piece we examined was how Islamists had co-opted and leveraged their own media in a more local setting (yet still networked to global audiences). Iraq was used as an illustrative example of how political Islamists were able to spread their virulent ideology by assuming control of a variety media outlets. Future means to help prevent future acquisition and exploitation of these media outlets by radical Islamists was also discussed.

What are lessons learned from this analysis of globalization and global media drivers of the Islamist Jihadist movement? Perhaps most importantly is that globalization and global media is a multi-faceted and complex system in today's world of technology and instant connectedness. There are, however, a there are a few things we might be able to accomplish in trying to contain and eventually reverse the growth of this Islamist movement. First, we need to assess the damage done in the recent past to the welfare state in the MENA region and look to ways to reimagine and reconstruct a viable return of the welfare state or a suitable sustainable replacement. Although there are virtues to capitalism, in certain areas of the world, MENA included, an unregulated market economy is likely to generate significant negative externalities. We need to work toward a capitalistic system that includes a compassionate dimension. Those who fall by the wayside of economic development have to fall into a safety net. Social welfare has to be that safety net. Government has to step up and provide social services effectively, universally, and equally to all citizens. What has become clear in the MENA region is that holes in the system are likely to be filled by social services run by Islamists. In turn, their acquired social power allows them to exploit that power for their own political and economic gain. Programs and social systems should be developed or adapted to discourage this Islamist political exploitation from happening.

Second, rampant consumerism should be better examined as to how it impacts disadvantaged and at-risk populations. Extremists and ideologues have historically exploited feeling of disenfranchisement and exclusion, both economic and social, for their own gain. A reimagining of sustainable and inclusive consumer marketplaces can potentially lead to a more efficient, but sustainable market that includes ethical consumption for its society. We need to further develop economic systems based around such things as Quality of Life and community well-being that do not only benefit individual consumers, but also pay respect to the society at large. Governments should also look to reform by working toward a system of regulations that would encourage business organizations to do more in terms of corporate social responsibility. We need to encourage cooperation between the profit and non-profit sectors to benefit society at large.

Third, we need to encourage media organizations, especially global media, to be more sensitive in their portrayals of Muslims and Islam in general. This is a critical piece and one that requires a multi-faceted approach that includes education as much as monitoring. Education programs can be developed to make media aware of the risks that certain programming and content might create. A Public–Private partnership can fund training program development and subsequent measurement methodologies. One will not be successful without the other. Once the program is in place monitoring programming content will help to better identify sources and outlets of concern and take corrective actions. The media landscape of the past is resplendent with examples of how media have become enlightened as to their negative portrayals of various groups and taken corrective action. One only needs to examine portrayals of women, African Americans, Gays and Lesbians, Latinos, Irish, etc. to see examples of the evolution and positive outcomes of enlightenment. The long and storied history of the Muslims offers a great many examples from which to choose positive characteristics of Muslims and Islam and avoid the negative stereotypes.

Fourth, international and national security organizations, as well as international NGO's dedicated to peace and social well-being, need to closely monitor the media landscape for propaganda from the extremist Islamist groups and counter this propaganda by images and argumentation that highlight the benefits of an inclusive society, a democratic society, a society that values cultural and religious diversity. Finally, we need to use all legal means possible to shut down media outlets used by terrorist organizations. We also should ensure that their toxic propaganda is not handed over to another media outlet to disseminate. May peace be on us all.

References

Abdel-Khalek, G. (1981). Looking outside, or turning Northwest? On the meaning and external dimension of Egypt's Infitah 1971–1980. *Social Problems, 28,* 394–408.

Ahmed, A. (1992). *Postmodernism and Islam: Predicament and promise.* London: Routledge.

Ahmed, A., & Donnan, H. (Eds.). (1994). *Islam, globalization, and postmodernity.* London: Routledge.

Allen, C., & Nielsen, J. (2002). *Summary report on Islamophobia in the EU after 11 September 2001.* Vienna, Austria: European Monitoring Centre on Racism and Xenophobia.

Al-Marashi, I. (2006/2007). *The dynamics of Iraqi's media: Ethno-sectarian violence, political Islam, public advocacy and globalization.* Central European University, Center for Policy Studies, Open Society Institute.

Al-Tamimi, A. J. (2014). The dawn of the Islamic State of Iraq and ash-Sham. *Current Trends in Islamist Ideology, 16,* 5–19.

Ayubi, N. (1991). *Political Islam: Religion and politics in the Arab World*. London and New York: Routledge.

Baker, R. W. (1981). Sadat's Open Door: Opposition from within. *Social Problems, 28,* 378–384.

Bardos, G. N. (2014). Jihad in the Balkans. *World Affairs, 177*(3), 73–79.

Beck, U. (1992). *Risk society: Toward a new modernity*. London: Sage Publications.

Brown, R. (2003). Spinning the war: Political communications, information operations and public diplomacy in the war on terrorism. In D. Kishan & D. Freedman (Eds.), *War and the Media* (p. 95). London: Sage.

Ciovacco, C. J. (2009). The contours of Al Qaeda's media strategy. *Studies in Conflict & Terrorism, 32*(10), 853–875.

Clark, J. (2004). Social movement theory and patron-clientelism: Islamic social institutions and the middle class in Egypt, Jordan, and Yemen. *Comparative Political Studies, 37*(8), 941–968.

Coll, S., & Glasser, S. B. (2005, August 7). Terrorists turn to the web as base of operations. *The Washington Post*.

Dessouki, A. E. (1981). Policy making in Egypt: A case study of the Open Door Economic Policy. *Social Problems, 28,* 410–416.

El-Aswad, E. (2013). Images of Muslims in Western scholarship and media after 9/11. *Digest of Middle East Studies (DOMES), 22*(1), 39–56.

El-Masry, M. (2002). *The future of Muslims in Canada*. Conference Paper October 20, 2002. Ottawa, Canada.

Esposito, J. (1992). *The Islamic threat, myth or reality*. New York and Oxford: Oxford University Press.

Fekete, L. (2002). *Racism: The hidden cost of September 11*. London: Institute of Race Relations.

Fucito, P. (2006). Al-Qaeda's media strategies. *Free EBooks Library, 5*.

Gellner, E. (1992). *Postmodernism, reason, and religion*. London: Routledge.

Howard, M. (2007, January 15). Insurgent TV channel turns into Iraq's newest cult hit. *The Guardian*. http://www.guardian.co.uk/Iraq/Story/0,,1990545,00.html.

Hunt, K. (2006, March 8). Osama Bin Laden fan clubs build online communities. *USA Today*.

Huntington, S. P. (1997). *The clash of civilizations and the remaking of world order*. India: Penguin Books.

Lane, D. (1999). Transformation of state socialism: From communism to chaotic capitalism. *Sociology, 33*(2), 447–450.

Lash, S., & Urry, J. (1987). *The end of organized capitalism*. Madison, WI: University of Wisconsin Press.

Lewis, B. (1990, September). Roots of Muslim rage. *Atlantic Monthly*.

Manning, P. (2006). Australians imagining Islam. In E. Poole & J. Richardson (Eds.), *Muslims and the news media* (pp. 128–141). London: I.B. Tauris.

McGeough, P. (2006a, February 14). On the Net: An open university for Jihad. *The Sydney Morning Herald*.

McGeough, P. (2006b, February 14). Death on film—Rebels wage war by video. *The Sydney Morning Herald*.

Muljadji, Y., Sekarningrum, B., & Muhammad, R. A. T. (2017). The Commodification of religious clothes through the social media: The identity crisis on youth Muslim female in urban Indonesia. *Romanian Journal of Journalism & Communication, 12*(2/3), 53–65.

Nye, J. S., Jr. (2004). *Soft power*. New York: Public Affairs.

Offe, C. (1985). *Disorganized capitalism: Contemporary transformations of work and politics*. Cambridge, MA: Polity Press.

Open Source Center. (2007). *Media aid: Iraq's Al-Zawra TV serves as insurgent propaganda vehicle*. Open Source Center (OSC) Media Aid, OSC Document: FEA20070202087288, December 17, 2006 to February 1, 2007.

Pipes, D. (2002). Islam and Islamism: Faith and ideology. *Policy: A Journal of Public Policy and Ideas, 18*(1), 22–26.

Poole, E., & Richardson, J. (Eds.). (2006). *Muslims and the news media*. London: I.B. Tauris.

Rawan, B., & Hussain, S. (2017). Reporting Ethnic Conflict in Karachi: Analysis through the Perspective of War and Peace Journalism. *Journal of Social Sciences & Humanities (1994–7046)*, *25*(2), 61–86.

Ronfeldt, D. (2005, March 2005). Al Qaeda and its affiliates: A global tribe waging segmental warfare. *First Monday*, p. 9. http://firstmonday.org/issues/issue10_3/ronfeldt/index.html.

Roy, O. (1994). *The failure of political Islam*. Cambridge, MA: Harvard University Press.

Sardar, Z., & Davies, M. W. (2002). *Why do people hate America?*. Cambridge, UK: Icon Books.

Saeed, A. (2004). 9/11 and the consequences for British-Muslims. In J. Morland & D. Carter (Eds.), *Anti-Capitalist Britain* (pp. 70–81). Manchester, UK: New Clarion Press.

Saeed, A. (2007). Media, racism and Islamophobia: The representation of Islam and Muslims in the media. *Sociology Compass, 1*(2), 443–462.

Schwartz, S. (2005). Radical Islam in America. *USA Today Magazine, 134*(2726), 16.

Shlapentokh, V. (2017). *A normal totalitarian society: How the Soviet Union functioned and how it collapsed*. London: Routledge.

Turner, B. S. (1994). *Orientalism, postmodernism, and globalism*. New York & London: Routledge.

Voll, J. O. (1994). *Islam: Continuity and change in the modern world*. New York: Syracuse University Press.

Zelizer, B., & Allan, S. (Eds.). (2002). *Journalism after 9/11*. London: Routledge.

Zubaida, S. (1993). *Islam, the people and the State: Political ideas and movements in the Middle East*. London: I.B. Tauris.

Chapter 7
Current Response: Counterterrorism Strategies Focusing on the Supply-Side of the Terrorism Market

Abstract Analysts have written copiously on ways to counteract radical Islam and Islamist militancy. Current public policy and counterterrorism strategies regarding Islamic militancy have focused mostly on short-term public safety, or what marketers may view as "supply-side" strategies. These are strategies designed to dismantle the marketing organization of militant Islamic groups. Supply-side strategies cannot effectively address the problem of radical Islam without developing compatible demand-side strategies—counterterrorism strategies designed to reduce demand. Thus, demand-side counterterrorism strategies serve to complement supply-side strategies. We try in this chapter to describe current terrorism policy and action focusing on the supply-side of the terrorism market.

Keywords Terrorism market · Counterterrorism · Supply-side strategies · Military force

7.1 Introduction

> Peace in the Middle East isn't going to be created by another war or violent act on the other side.
>
> Mandy Patinkin[1]

> If we destroy human rights and rule of law in the response to terrorism, they have won.
>
> Joichi Ito[2]

Let us begin by saying that the military power that can be brought to bear from Western powers is overwhelmingly superior to anything that the terrorists can counter with (short of obtaining nuclear weaponry). Our application of this power, whether in the support of ground units taking territory or surgical strikes to decimate Islamist

---

[1] https://www.brainyquote.com/quotes/mandy_patinkin_591599.
[2] https://www.brainyquote.com/quotes/joichi_ito_206748.

© Springer Nature Switzerland AG 2019
M. J. Sirgy et al., *Combatting Jihadist Terrorism through Nation-Building*, Human Well-Being Research and Policy Making, https://doi.org/10.1007/978-3-030-17868-0_7

leadership has been substantial. At the same time, we have applied a variety of intelligence gathering and monitoring programs in these regions. These programs run the gamut from the technology based types of monitoring and gathering intel like signals intelligence (SIGINT), imagery intelligence (IMINT), measurement and signature intelligence (MASINT), to the human side (HUMIT).[3] In the age of technology, the value of the final one of these, HUMIT, was marginalized to varying degrees by governments and military brass. Networks on the ground of nations facing rising Islamist movements, that had been built at a great cost in blood and treasure were either disbanded or simply "left to wither on the vine." This marginalization of HUMIT let the intensity and size of the Islamist terror movements in several areas of perceived "pacified ground" rise with a vengeance. This left Western powers and the local institutions they supported without necessary amounts of information and its correct interpretations to make effective and timely interdictions. Hence, decisions were, at times, based on flawed cultural intelligence. That is, responses to the threat were planned and executed at times by individuals guilty of ethnocentric interpretations, or so-called "mirror-imaging (see Heuer, 1999). This flawed understanding of information and intelligence can also exist between indigenous country leaders of the elite urban class and the more local peoples of given agrarian or even urban environments. A more general Western population example of errant interpretations is below.

Many Westerners may believe that the founders of al-Qaeda and ISIS are religious fundamentalists; this is not necessarily the case. The jihadist organizations are more political than religious entities. Some scholars refer to Islamist terrorist groups as "Islamo-Leninists" because these groups have a utopian-totalitarian vision. This vision is best articulated by Ayman al-Zawahiri, al-Qaeda's chief ideologist, who espouses the group as a force or a vanguard designed to mobilize Muslims across the globe to rise up against their corrupt rulers, who are in power because of the corrupt Western powers who support these rulers (Friedman, 2007; Martin, 2018). Muslims then should work to overthrow these secular rulers through a corrupted ideal of jihad based on the premise that they defile Islam. According to this canon, corrupt regimes should be replaced by Islamic regimes reflective of the Caliphate rule from the height of the Islamic empire. A supreme religious-political leader, similar to a Caliph, would unite all Muslims into a single community.

The purpose of this chapter is to describe current counterterrorism policies and action by Western and non-Western governments. We approach the subject matter from what some would call an economics, or perhaps a marketing, perspective. Political scientists and sociologists have written considerably on Islamic militancy (e.g., Ali & Post, 2008; Wiktorowicz & Kaltenthaler, 2006), and the topic is covered in the fields of anthropology (Asad, 2007; el-Aswad, 2012, 2013; Hefner, 2002), history (e.g., Lincoln, 2006), management (e.g., Bell, 2002), economics (e.g., Shughart II, 2006), international business (e.g., Larobina & Pate, 2009), psychology (e.g., Crowson, Debacker, & Thoma, 2006), law (e.g., Berman, 2006), and international studies (e.g., Munson, 2004), among other disciplines.

---

[3] AAP-6 (2004)—NATO Glossary of terms and definitions.

Historically, marketing scholars have shied away from this topic, perhaps because they do not see it as within the scope of marketing. This view may be shared by some scholars from other disciplines. However, radical Islam can be treated as a "lethal" market, in the manner that social marketers and macromarketers previously treated other socially undesirable phenomena such as drug abuse (e.g., Smith & Fitchett, 2002), cigarette smoking (e.g., Comm, 1997; Wall, 2005), excessive drinking (e.g. Wall, 2005, 2006), unsafe sex and the spread of STDs (e.g., Haq et al., 2011), wasting energy (e.g., Frisble, 1980; Harvey & Kerin, 1977), littering and polluting (e.g., Bagozzi & Dabholkar, 1994), the overuse and abuse of the automobile (e.g., Wall, 2005, 2006; Wright & Eagan, 2000), overuse of healthcare services (e.g., Borkowsk, 1994), the illegal purchase of firearms (Gundlach, Bradford & Wilkie, 2010), among others.

These "lethal" markets prove difficult to eliminate but may be reduced through what is referred to as "demarketing." We believe that a supply/demand approach to combating Islamic militancy based on demarketing is likely to be more effective than fragmented approaches that focus on short-term public safety. Adopting a demarketing approach to radical Islam (Kotler & Levy, 1971) should prompt counterterrorism experts and public policy officials to focus on the "big picture," which in essence involves a market-based problem. The demarketing approach focuses on both supply- and demand-side strategies of counterterrorism. Supply-side strategies focus on understanding the marketing organization of Islamist militancy and systematically deducing demarketing strategies related to the various marketing and human resource management elements and sub-elements. In essence, supply-side strategies are short-term strategies designed to dismantle existing militant organizations. However, supply-side strategies are not likely to prevent the re-emergence of future militant organizations. To combat such re-emergence, we need to apply demand-side strategies (i.e., designed to address the problem in a long-term horizon). Demand-side strategies are deduced from a thorough analysis of the environment that promote the emergence (or re-emergence) of militant organizations—environmental factors such as changes in the economic, political, religious, globalization, media, and cultural conditions.[4] This is what we have done in the preceding chapters—to focus on combatting terrorism through nation building. Strategies associated with nation building (i.e., a quality-of-life approach) focus on the demand side of the market equation. This chapter complements the preceding chapters by focusing on the supply side of the equation.

7.2 Supply-Side Counterterrorism Policies and Action: Dismantling the Islamist Jihadist Organization

Supply-side counterterrorism strategies focus on the dismantling of the marketing organization of Islamic militancy. To help the reader understand counterterrorism

---

[4]For demand-side strategies of counterterrorism, see Chap. 8.

Table 7.1 The marketing elements of radical Islam militant organization

		Radical Islamist marketing
Market		Muslims across the global, especially devout Muslims
Functional service offering		Gaining status and prominence in the political and global stage using violent means to quell infidels (and Muslims allied with infidels)
Emotional service offering		Providing a channel for the release of cultural and religious anger and grievance
Marketing management	Goals and objectives	Striving to achieve a certain level of awareness of the terrorists' cause, justifying terrorist action, developing a favorable attitude toward the terrorist cause, raising funds, and recruiting new members
	Product strategy	Acquiring arms and WMD, planning terrorist operations, and executing these operations
	Price strategy	Using narcotic trade and money laundering schemes to finance the terrorist operations
	Place strategy	Selecting sites of terrorist operations and transporting terrorists and arms (WMD) to these sites to implement planned operations
	Promotion strategy	Promoting the terrorist cause using the Internet, educational institutions, and opinion leaders
Human resources management	Goals and objectives	Striving to increase membership of terrorist agents to man planned operations and enhance loyalty and commitment of agents to the organization and cause
	Recruiting of agents	Recruiting Muslim youth to conduct terrorist operations
	Training of agents	Training recruits to conduct terrorist operations
	Motivating the agents	Motivating the trained recruits for terrorist operations

policies in place, we need to set the stage by describing a typical marketing organization of Islamic militancy. Islamist militant organizations employ agents to provide a political service. These organizations are designed to assist Muslims in political transactions with infidels and other Muslims who are allied with infidels. As such, this is the *market* of radical Islam militant organizations (see Table 7.1).

What is the *service offered* by Islamist militant organizations? These marketing organizations offer a service that meets market demand. The service involves both functional and emotional dimensions. The functional service includes the use of various violent means to quell infidels and/or Muslims allied with infidels (e.g., suicide bombings, assassinations of political figure heads, attacking military installations, abductions and ransom demands, beheadings, roadside bombings, attacking heavily populated civilian sites, demolishing key cultural sites, and acquiring and using weapons of mass destruction). The emotional service offering provides a channel for the release of the cultural and religious anger and grievance against infidels and others for perceived cultural and religious affronts.

Knowing what the market and service offerings of Islamist militant organizations are, we now can turn to understanding the various elements of marketing management and human resources management inherent in those organizations.

7.2.1 The Marketing Management System of Jihadist Organizations and Counterterrorism Strategies

We begin by identifying the marketing goals and objectives of Islamist militant organizations. These may include the following:

- Increase awareness of the emotional mission of Islamist militant organization XYZ in the minds of the Muslim population,
- Instill a belief in the minds of the Muslim population that *jihad* (political violence against infidels and allies of infidels) is the only means to restore Islamic hegemony in the world,
- Strive to have a significant segment of the Muslim population to form a positive impression of the organization, and
- Strive to recruit a significant segment of the Muslim population to join the movement and/or contribute resources.

Understanding how Islamist militant organizations market themselves requires an understanding of how they apply the basic four "P's" of marketing strategies: (1) product strategy (i.e., selecting terrorist methods, planning and conducting operations), (2) price strategy (i.e., identify and pursue funding sources, setting up a financial system to receive funds, laundering money, and funding militant operations), (3) place strategy (i.e., select locations for operations and transport recruits and material to those locations), and (4) promotion strategy (e.g., promotion to recruit militants, raise funds, and influence public opinion). Understanding the business of marketing of Islamist militancy could help the reader better understand the counterterrorism policies in place.

The Product Element: To reiterate, the goals of these radical Jihadist organizations can be articulated as: increase public awareness of the terrorist cause, instill beliefs that terrorist action is justified, develop a favorable attitude toward the cause, and increase membership. As such product strategy of an Islamist militancy organization would typically involve three major elements to achieve organizational goals: (1) the planning of terrorist operations, (2) the execution of these operations, and (3) the acquisition of weapons of mass destruction.

The *planning of terrorist operations* (e.g., suicide bombings, assassination of political figure heads, abductions and ransom demands, roadside bombings, etc.) may not necessarily be formulated by the radical Muslim clerics, the recruiters, or the trainers. Typically, there is a person who plays the role of the "mastermind" of planned operations. For example, Khalid Sheikh Mohammed has been accused of masterminding the September 11 attacks. He is not a cleric, not a recruiter, nor is he a trainer.[5] Counterterrorism officials counteract the planning of terrorist operations by identifying and arrest the mastermind behind the planned operations. This means good intelligence, the sharing of intelligence with law enforcement officials, and the efficient and prompt response of law enforcement to intelligence. Once arrested, accused masterminds are interrogated to identify the exact militants involved and act to foil further terrorists' action.

Once a terrorist operation is underway, counterterrorism officials work closely with local law enforcement agencies to ensure that likely target facilities of attack are well-secured and people in these facilities are highly vigilant of suspicious behavior, as is typically done in airports around the globe. Of course, such a tactic is commonly used but is also criticized by many social scientists. Such heightened vigilantism breeds lack of trust (Ersen, 2007; Ghaffarzadegan, 2008). Counterterrorism officials typically use the alert system (such as the one implemented in airports).

Counterterrorism agencies tend to coordinate with local law enforcement agencies to foil terrorist action. This is especially true when the counterterrorism action takes place in a Muslim country, not on Western soil. In other words, Western counterterrorism agencies tend to support Muslim governments in their attempt to combat terrorism, to avoid taking over the fighting. Taking over the fighting tends to further polarize the feeling of "us against them" about non-Muslim interference—polarization tend to further unite Muslims and turn moderate Muslims into radical ones (Huntington, 1993, 1996). See Box 7.1 for an example of the use of drones and its collateral damage.

Box 7.1: The Pros and Cons of Using Drones in Counterterrorism Operations

In 2011, president Obama ordered the targeting and remote control assassination of Anwar al-Awlaki, a Yemen-based American jihadi terrorist. Up to 2011, Awlaki managed to recruit many jihadi militants and plot the mass killing of American citizens for al-Qaeda.

After the successful assassination of al-Awlaki, the use of drones seems to have been elevated as an anti-terrorism weapon of choice. Drone strikes were used repeatedly by the Obama administration as well as the Trump administration. What is the net effect of drones? On the positive side, if drones were to have been used to assassinate the plotters of 9/11/2001, such use could have saved 3000 from dying. As such, one can appreciate drones as a panacea of sorts. In contrast, the use of drones can further alienate and radicalize moderate Muslims in the long run. Drone use then could be deemed to be, in the long term, more detrimental than helpful in mitigating Islamist terrorism.

Adapted from International Peace Institute (2016).

---

[5]http://en.wikipedia.org/wiki/Khalid_Sheikh_Mohammed.

The *acquisition of weapons of mass destruction* (WMD) is a subject of great concern for not only counterterrorism officials but of national security and foreign policy. The threat of terrorism is exponentially multiplied by the access of terrorists to WMD's. The United States, Great Britain, and their allies went to war against Iraq over repeated violations of UN sanctions and concerns about WMDs. The United Nations International Atomic Energy Agency (IAEA) has been hard at work monitoring the development of nuclear energy and its potential conversion to WMS. Much of the international community is in uproar over Iran's use of nuclear fuel. Similarly, North Korea has been generally considered a pariah by the international community for its nuclear armaments. One can view all the efforts of the IAEA and the many sanctions imposed by the international community on states that have violated the nonproliferation treaty.

What is troubling—besides the fact that countries such as Iran have the capability of developing WMD—is the notion that WDM can be acquired (or purchased) on the black market. Of course, there are many instances of counterterrorism efforts related to the acquisition of WMD. For example, in 2003, the U.S. Government has led several multinational initiatives such as the Global Partnership against the Spread of WMD, the *Global Threat Reduction Initiative*, and the *Proliferation Security Initiative* (PSI) (Speier, Chow, & Starr, 2001). In regard to the latter (PSI), this initiative was a global effort designed to stop the trafficking of WMD, their delivery systems, and related materials to and from states and non-states worldwide. In 2004, the Security Council adopted *Resolution 1540* that requires all UN member states to refrain from providing support to non-state actors that attempt to develop or acquire WMD and their means of delivery. The UN General Assembly followed suit in 2005—the assembly adopted the *Convention on the Suppression of Acts of Nuclear Terrorism* (Nuclear Terrorism Convention). Furthermore, in late 2005, US Department of State created the Office of Weapons of Mass Destruction Terrorism. The mission of this new agency is work with domestic and international partners to develop and implement strategies to prevent, protect against, and respond to the threat or use of WMD by terrorists.[6]

The Price Element: The price element involves identifying and securing funds for terrorist operations (e.g., revenue from the narcotic trade and money laundering). Let's begin this discussion by first focusing on *revenues from the narcotic trade* that are used to finance terrorist operations. In 1999, the *International Convention for the Suppression of the Financing of Terrorism* was adopted in the United Nations General Assembly. The law is designed to facilitate the prosecution of persons accused of involvement in the financing of terrorist activities by forcing country signatories to extradite the accused to trial purposes. In 2005, the Council of Europe introduced *The Council of Europe Convention on Laundering, Search, Seizure and Confiscation of the Proceeds from Crime and the Financing of Terrorism*, which is an application of UN convention (Klein, 2009).

Narco-terrorism is a worldwide phenomenon. In a report delivered before the U.S. House Committee on the Judiciary Subcommittee on Crime, countless exam-

---

[6]www.state.gov/documents/organization/65477.pdf.

ples narco-Islamist terrorism was provided in Europe (e.g., Kosovo and Turkey), Middle East (e.g., Lebanon), Central Asia (e.g., Chechnya), South and East Asia (e.g., Philippines), and so on. A pointed example is the source of revenue for the Taliban. It was estimated that 80% of revenue raised for Taliban fighters is derived from the narcotic trade (Cillufo, 2000). Afghanistan generates 75% of the world's opiates.

Counterterrorism policies in this instance entail the strengthening of domestic legal institutions and social organizations in afflicted countries. It also entails developing a set of outreach programs from these institutions to individuals and smaller villages in the agrarian regions and to neighborhoods in urban areas. As noted at the beginning of this chapter developing local HUMIT is a key to understanding the various needs and wants of the given populations. This structure ultimately means aiding the afflicted countries carry out effective law enforcement through supporting the development of a well-developed "marketing research" program at the local and state levels that would lead to the successful identification of and ultimate removal of terrorists. A removal that would be viewed in a positive light by the locals in either the urban or agrarian marketplace. In other words, military efforts to fight narco-terrorists must be complemented with domestic policies that reach down to the local level that ultimately serve to buttress law enforcement and the judicial system in the countries where the terrorists raise revenue to finance their terrorist action (Cillufo, 2000; Sagan, 2004).

Now, let us focus on *money laundering*. To operate on a global scale, Islamist militant organizations deposit, withdraw, and transfer money through banking. The Islamist vast majority of banks worldwide have specific policies and safeguards designed to rule out investments and money laundering associated with terrorist activities. Counterterrorism policies related to money laundering of Islamist militancy vary considerably (Bjorklund, Reynoso, & Hazlett, 2005; Pieth, 2006). For example, the International Monetary Fund (IMF) a 34-member inter-government agency established by the 1989 G-7 Summit in Paris in cooperation with the World Bank, called the *Financial Action Task Force on Money Laundering* (FATF), works closely with other key international organizations to implement anti-money laundering programs worldwide.[7] Part of the *US Patriot Act*, adopted in response to September 11, 2001 terrorist attacks, is designed to strengthen U.S. measures to prevent, detect, and prosecute money laundering that helps finance Islamic militancy.[8] Furthermore, the US Department of Treasury has developed a set of guidelines for public accountants to identify money laundering activities and to report such activities[9] (Abuza, 2003).

The Place Element: The Place element of Islamist militant organizations is essentially the selection of location and sites for militant operations in ways to achieve the maximum terrorist impact. Another element of the place strategy is the transport of recruits and weapon material to sites of operations.

---

[7]http://www.imf.org/external/np/exr/facts/aml.htm.

[8]http://www.fincen.gov/statutes_regs/files/hr3162.pdf.

[9]http://www.ustreas.gov/offices/enforcement/money_laundering.shtml.

With respect to the *selection of location and sites for militant operations*, good intelligence is key to effective counterterrorism. Again, as noted above, the need for a well-supported integrated intelligence system that links both forward and backward exchange of relevant and timely credible information is crucial. For example, intelligence was able to detect specific communication that hinted at New York City being target of several terrorist plots.[10] Intelligence that help alert counterterrorism officials of specific target sites help secure these sites.

Now let's turn to *transportation of terrorists and shipment of WMD*. There are many counterterrorism policies in place. For example, the US Transportation Security Administration (TSA) have policies designed to detect Islamist terrorists in air transit. These policies are highly varied: from imaging, luggage restrictions, profiling, to observation of irregular behavior. For example, Logan International Airport enhanced security by using a behavior pattern recognition program. Security personnel are trained to observe and interview passengers and others and identify Islamic militants accordingly. The vast majority of airports worldwide have followed suit (U.S. Department of Homeland Security, 2011).

Another counterterrorism strategy related to transportation is holding governments accountable to secure their own borders. A case in point was the argument that was made regarding Islamist militants were infiltrating the Mexican borders to enter and reach target sites in the U.S. (Helms, 2009). In the MENA, border security played a role when al-Qaeda fighters infiltrated the Syrian borders into Iraq to conduct suicide missions. Counterterrorism in this instance tend to be in the form of putting pressure on governments to police their own borders and holding them accountable when infiltrations occur (Glon, 2005).

Another place element is the *shipment and delivery of arms* for specific terrorist operations, especially WMD. In parallel, counterterrorism efforts focus on identifying the types of arms typically used in terrorist operations (especially WMD), track the sources of supply, and intercept shipments. A good example of interception of arms shipment to terrorist groups was seen when the Israeli Navy was able to capture a ship carrying a large shipment of weapons (including rockets, motor shells, and anti-tank weapons) from Iran. The arms shipment was destined to Hezbollah fighters in Lebanon (Intelligence and Terrorism Information Center, 2009). For this interception to have occurred Israeli counterterrorism officials must have had good, local HUMIT intelligence regarding the arm shipment and the specific transportation route related to that shipment. The lesson to be learned is have intelligence regarding the types of arms used by Islamist militants, the source of these arms, the destination of the shipment, and the shipment route. Intelligence gathering is again one of creating a fully integrated system that also gives locals an impetus to aid in the reduction and destruction of the terrorism activities and organizations themselves.

The Promotion Element: The Promotion element of the marketing of Islamist militancy involves three principal elements: (a) the use of the Internet and mobile media to propagate the terrorist cause, (c) the use of educational institutions to impress youth and raise funds, and (c) the use Muslim clerics as opinion leaders.

---

[10]http://www.cbsnews.com/video/watch/?id=7382308n.

Let us first focus on the *use of the Internet and mobile media*. Radical Islamist groups have managed to promote their cause on the Internet and receive contributions through charity-type organizations. For example, Hamas is considered by many in the Islamic world to be a charity organization whose mission is to help impoverished Palestinians. Syria plays host to many Hamas officials. Hamas has many of its offices in the Damascus.[11] A report by Homeland Security has documented that there is a great deal of evidence pointing to the increasingly large role the Internet plays in promoting Islamist militancy (U.S. Department of Homeland Security, 2009). The report coined the Internet as a "radicalization accelerant." The report cites evidence indicating that in 1980 there were 12 terrorist-related websites. By 2003 this number grew to 2630 sites, and by January 2009 that number exploded to 6940 sites. The use of the internet by radical Islamist groups is widespread not only in MENA and the West, but also is targeting the largest Muslim country in the world, Indonesia. Indonesia has historically been a very secular oriented Muslim society. As noted in an earlier chapter, the impact on facilitating a more radical view of Islam by these Islamist "marketers" is significant. Messages are tailored to local culture and narratives to influence the acceptance of the message and the "product" (Hui, 2010).

Here are some examples of counterterrorism policies related to the use of the Internet to counteract the use of Jihadist promotion. Counterterrorism officials have launched persuasion campaigns targeting moderate Muslim officials and influential religious figures to address fallacies and distortions propagated by the radical Jihadist organizations, and that these counterterrorism messages were disseminated through the Internet (McCulloch, 2005). Other counterterrorism measures include reaching out to the vulnerable youth where they are online (e.g., social networking sites and interactive video streaming sites) to inoculate youth against radical Jihadist propaganda. There were instances in which counterterrorism agents and agencies took advantage of the viral nature of online content (e.g., using "viral" marketing to facilitate and encourage people to pass along the counter attitudinal message) (Bahgat, 2004; Karmon, 2007). At the same time, Muslim users of the internet have moved the Muslim discussion forward on their own. Recent work shows how Islamic emoji use by younger Sunni Muslims has opened up a wide ranging discussion of Muslim interpretations and taking personal control of Muslim issues of identity and such Stanton (2018).

How about the *use of educational institutions* to propagate the radical Jihadist message? Hamas has managed to do much promotion and raise much money through their education center, Al Maghrib.[12] The center conducts Islamic knowledge seminars and through its website it encourages visitors to donate money. As of 2003 US intelligence sources estimated that Hamas had an annual budget of 50 million dollars, raining much of this money through its reputation as a charity organization.[13]

Recruiting of Islamic militants typically occurs by recruiters working in concert with radical Muslim clerics (i.e., *opinion leaders*). That is, recruiting is typically

---

[11] http://www.globalsecurity.org/military/world/para/hamas-funds.htm.

[12] http://www.jihadwatch.org/2009/05/us-muslim-website-raising-money-for-hamas.html.

[13] http://www.globalsecurity.org/military/world/para/hamas-funds.htm.

local and associated with Muslim studies. Consider the following case in London. The Queen's Road mosque in Walthamstow, northeast London is run by Tabilighi Jamaat. This cleric has very severe fundamental views of Islam and Islamic Jihad and an emotional connection with his congregation. The militants who conducted the fertilizer bomb attack of 2004, and the July 7 and July 21 bombings of 2005 in London, were all recruited from that mosque. Others were recruited at British colleges (O'Neill, 2009). It has been also noted that mosques, universities and charities are the nodes where al-Qaeda's recruiters seek new members (Gerwehr & Daly, 2006).

Counterterrorism action has been directed to offset recruiting conducted mostly in mosques and institutions of higher education. This has been done mostly through intelligence gathering to identify recruiters in mosques and institutions of higher learning. Once these recruiters are identified, counterterrorist agents have made every attempt to dissuade them from this activity by applying a mix of persuasion and legal techniques. In other words, if persuasive techniques fail, counterterrorism officials often resort to arrest and prosecution (Djerejian et al., 2003; Kelman, 1961; Post, 2007).

7.2.2 The Human Resources Management System of Jihadist Organizations and Counterterrorism Strategies

What would be the human resources management goals and objectives of Islamist militant organizations? These may include the following:

- Increase membership of terrorist agents to ensure quality and quantity manpower to carry out planned terrorist operations, and
- Increase commitment and loyalty to the Islamist militant organization and the cause at large.

There is a fair amount of literature regarding the use of Islamic principles in Human Resource Management (Rana & Malik, 2016; Samier 2017; Zangoueinezhad & Moshabaki, 2011). To begin to understand how Islamist militant organizations operate intelligence gathering should begin with the review of the existing literature on Islamic HR. It is logical, that Islamist militant organizations would at least follow a framework and application based on these principles. It clearly would involve more information given the output being radical terrorism, but the foundation would be expected to be useful for interpretation. Understanding how Islamic militant organizations manage to achieve their human resources goals and objectives in term of recruitment, training, compensating and motivating radical Muslim youth is key to counterterrorism strategies.

The Recruitment Element: Recruitment strategy of an Islamist militant organization may involve (1) the analysis of the physical/intellectual/emotional/social characteristics of selected terrorist agents, (2) selection of agents from a larger pool of recruits, and (3) evaluation of the recruitment procedure based on the success or failure of past militant operations. Based on such analysis, counterterrorism strategies designed to undermine the recruitment element of radical jihadist organizations can be identified and detailed.

The recruitment of Islamist militants is typically conducted in mosques by recruiters directly associated with Muslim clerics (Cillufo, 2000; Laquer, 2000; Naipal, 1982). As such, counterterrorism agencies spend much time, effort, and money gathering intelligence of mosques that have radical clerics. The goal is to neutralize these clerics and their cadres of recruiters by legal and persuasion means (McCauley & Moskalenko, 2011; Post, 2007). In other words, all means of persuasion are used to dissuade radical clerics from using violence and the pursuit of armed struggle. Legal means (e.g., incarceration) is also used. Gerwehr and Daly (2006) suggested that Islamism's opponents ought to rely less on a handful of liberal clerics and instead stitch together a broad anti-Islamist coalition of secularists, moderate Muslims, business elites, women's groups and the military. Open debate among moderate and radical Muslim clerics is encouraged to deliver this message. Counterterrorism officials encourage open debate through a variety of public and private forums (e.g., Centre for Islamic Studies in Queens Village, New York), centers of Islamic studies in educational institutions (e.g., The King Fahd Center for Middle East and Islamic Studies; Oxford Centre for Islamic Studies in Oxford, United Kingdom in Arkansas, USA), Muslim-type of educational institutions (e.g., University of Al-Qarawiyyin in Morocco, Al-Azhar University in Cairo, Al-Mustansiriya University in Baghdad), as well as in some "madrassas" around the globe (e.g., Jamia Nizamia in Hyderabad, India; Jam'iah Arabia Ashan ul Uloom in Gulshan-e-Iqbal, Karachi, India; Al-Imaan University in Riydah, Saudi Arabia).

The Training Element: The training of terrorists requires trainers, facilities, organization, and funding. The former Iraqi regime of Saddam Hussein trained thousands of Islamist terrorists in camps in Iraq over many years preceding the U.S. invasion (Hayes, 2006). Intelligence has provided the military and other international and national law enforcement agencies with information about possible location of training facilities of al-Qaeda, ISIS, and other Islamist militant groups. For example, Indian intelligence identified al-Qaeda militant training located in Afghanistan and Pakistan around the time of the September 11, 2001 attacks—over 120 training camps (Bindra, 2001). According to Israeli authorities, a terrorist training camp requires a logistical support infrastructure of upwards of 20 persons, including quartermasters and trainers. The larger the operation, the more opportunities exist to identify the participants and disrupt it (Karmon, 2007). Of course, the counterterrorism policy here is to identify and dismantle the training facilities.

But what can counterterrorism agents and agencies do with the trainers? In many instances the trainers are likely to make a living and receive financial remuneration for their work. For some, radical jihad is just a job. Although there is no direct correlation between low GDP and terrorism, poor people in countries with high levels of unemployment are more vulnerable to recruitment (Stern, 2010). If the funding stops, so does the training. To ensure that the trainers do not seek similar opportunities, counterterrorism officials assist potential trainers in finding suitable employment opportunities.

What happens, however, when the trainers are also radical in their belief system? Evidence shows how the mindset of terrorists turns into a belief system after joining a terrorist organization (Eren, 2007). Counterterrorism agents can use similar promotion methods to change the attitude of the trainers (Post, 2007).

The most successful rehabilitation models focus on the motivations of individual offenders (Stern, 2010). The ideal approach includes three components. Each of the three is crucial to the ultimate success of the program. The components are: prison-based rehabilitation programs, services to help released prisoners reintegrate into society, and post-release services. The local community's involvement in the post-release services, in particular, seems essential to reducing recidivism rates. Although terrorists are different from ordinary criminals in many ways, it is worth noting that according to the Saudi government, its de-radicalization program with the three-step approach mentioned above has been extraordinarily successful. According to official statistics, the rate of recidivism is 10–20%, far lower than that for ordinary criminals. The most successful rehabilitation models focus on the motivations of individual offenders (Robertson & Cruickshank, 2009; Stern, 2010).

Counterterrorism officials take additional measures to prevent terrorist training camps from being re-occupied for the same purpose. One measure seems to be the building of schools and educational institutions at former terrorist training sites (Huntington, 1993, 1996). Why? Training sites for extremists are not built and operated in a vacuum. The social, cultural, economic, and political surroundings facilitate the development of these training camps. Operating Western-style educational institutions seems to be an effective means to alter the social, cultural, economic, and political landscape of the region. That is, providing social value in education within an additional context of being an education that is more tolerant to Western values may be an effective means to prevent the return of Islamist extremists to the region.

The Motivation and Compensation Element: Typically, militants who are being prepared to conduct terrorist operations are placed in a social network that provides them the strong moral support for their planned action. In other words, they may be isolated from people who may object to the impending operation and possibly risk foiling the operation (National Commission on Terrorist Attacks upon the United States, 2004). To counteract this phase of the operation, intelligence is gathered to identify the safe havens where the militants are being prepared for the planned terror attacks. It has long been recognized that intelligence is at the heart of countering terrorism (Sloan, 2002). This again points to the critical nature of local, on the ground, HUMIT as outlined at the beginning of this chapter. Counterterrorism officials use intelligence in at least two ways to foil planned operations. One is the use of force to eliminate the threat. The other is by providing information to family members about the planned operations. In most cases family members are not likely to be extremists in their views (McCauley & Moskalenko, 2011). The aftermath of terrorist operations usually brings deep shame and humiliation on the family. In many cases there is retribution against family members. Therefore, there is a strong motive for family members to prevent terrorist operations and given a chance they tend to locate the suspects and take measures to foil the planned operations.

It should be noted that Saddam Hussein recognized the shame and humiliation experienced by families of Palestinians who engaged in terrorist attacks against Israelis. To prevent family members from intervening and foiling terrorist operations against Israelis, he established a support program in which families of so-called Palestinian martyrs were compensated to the tune of US$ 10–25,000. Such financial support added a new dimension of legitimacy to the martyrdom cause and served to diffuse resistance of family members.[14] Judiciously applied, the same tactic is commonly used by counterterrorism officials to ensure the support of family members against target suspects.

Counterterrorism officials will also use a fully Integrated Marketing Communications (IMC) campaign using advertising and other media directed to the general public in a nation or more local municipality or village. A typical campaign depicts terrorists in negative terms, profiling them, and warning the public to be on the lookout for such individuals. Such advertising has been run by government agencies with assistance from the U.S. State Department (Fullerton & Kendrick, 2006; Peter, Bloomgarden, & Grunwald, 2003; Skuba, 2002; Tuch, 1990).

7.3 Conclusion

While research has shown a positive shift in Muslim public perceptions in different indicators that relate to extremist positions and terrorism, it is important to remember that moderates and extremists share perceptions on many issues and that the extremist minority is still a large group.

A fundamental requirement for any Western effort to communicate with Muslim audiences, whether it be through diplomacy, media reporting, or marketing, is to begin with an attitude of respect and open-mindedness that is free of ethnocentrism and stereotypical thinking. Understanding the overlapping attitudes shared by extremists and moderates is essential for any communications to be effective. Based on a Pew Research Center study, there were 1.8 billion Muslims as of 2015, roughly 24% of the world's population (Lipka, 2017). If the 7 percent of the politically radicalized continue to feel politically dominated, occupied, and disrespected, the West will have little, if any, chance of changing their minds (Esposito & Mogahed, 2007). This is a hypothetical idea not a tested or documented fact.

Combating terrorism using military force to dismantle radical Islamist organizations can be viewed as supply-side counterterrorism. This chapter identified a variety of supply-side counterterrorism strategies commonly used by Western and non-Western governments. These are summarized in Table 7.2. We also hope that public policy officials who are focused on counterterrorism would find the framework we used in this chapter helpful in further guiding their decision-making.

---

[14]http://www.foxnews.com/story/0,2933,48822,00.html.

Table 7.2 Summary of supply-side counterterrorism policies in place

Major goals	Specific counterterrorism policies in place
Undermine the terrorist organization's marketing management goals of • Increasing Arabs and Muslims' awareness of the terrorists' cause, • Impressing Arabs and Muslims that terrorist action is justified, • Fostering a favorable attitude among Arabs and Muslims toward the cause, and • Encouraging Arabs and Muslims to become members of their organizations and contribute resources	**Product** • Identifying and arresting the "mastermind" of terrorist plots • Alerting local officials to protect individuals and institutions that are targets of terrorist plots • Curbing the distribution of WMD on the black market
	Price • Cracking down on the narcotics trade that finances terrorism • Curbing money laundering connected to terrorist organizations
	Place • Identifying potential target sites of terrorist plots • Using equipment and technology to spot terrorists in transit • Encouraging individual countries to secure their own borders to prevent terrorist infiltration • Intercepting potential shipment of terrorist arms, especially WMD
	Promotion • Identifying and shutting down Internet websites directly and indirectly used by terrorist organizations to promote their cause • Identifying and neutralizing key radical Muslim clerics and other opinion leaders directly or indirectly involved in promoting the terrorists' cause
Undermining the terrorist organization's human resource management goals of increasing the cadre of terrorist agents and enhancing their loyalty and commitment to the terrorist organization and the radical Jihad cause at large	**HR-recruitment** • Identifying and neutralizing terrorist recruiters directly or indirectly involved in recruiting new members
	HR-training • Identifying and dismantling terrorist training facilities • Identifying terrorist trainers by motive (money versus ideology); trainers motivated by money are assisted to make a living in other occupations that are legitimate; trainers motivated by ideology are subjected to de-radicalization programs • Replacing terrorist training facilities with Western-type educational institutions
	HR-motivation and compensation • Families of terrorist agents are persuaded to rein in their terrorist family member(s) • Alerting the general public, particularly in the Arab and Muslim world, of the dangers of terrorism and specific terror suspects

Table 7.3 Policies and programs related to counterterrorism

Policy	Rationale	Objectives	Resources
Use of force	Symbolic strength	Punish or destroy the terrorists	Military and paramilitary assets (punitive and preemptive strikes); covert operations (use of special forces)
Legalistic options	Rule of law	International cooperation; prosecution, conviction, and incarceration of terrorists	International organizations; law enforcement agencies; domestic legal establishments
Operations other than war: Repressive options	Deterrence; prediction; destabilization	Disruption of the terrorists; intelligence; coercion of supporters	Technologies; intelligence operatives; covert operations
Operations other than war: Conciliatory options	Resolve underlying problems	End immediate crises; forestall future crises	Diplomacy; social reform; economic assets; negotiations and concessions

Source Adapted from Martin (2018, p. 359)

Table 7.3 outlines a categorization of policies and programs of counterterrorism. Note that the first three rows (use of force, legalistic options, operations other than war—repressive options) are all supply-side counterterrorism strategies. The last row (operations other than war—conciliatory options) hint at demand-side counterterrorism measures to which Chap. 8 discusses in some detail.

References

Abuza, Z. (2003). Funding terrorism in Southeast Asia: The financial network of Al Qaeda and Jemaah Islamiya. *Contemporary Southeast Asia: A Journal of International and Strategic Affairs, 25*(2), 169–199.

Asad, T. (2007). *On suicide bombing.* New York: Columbia University Press.

Ali, F., & Post, J. (2008). The history and evolution of martyrdom in the service of defensive Jihad: An analysis of suicide bombers in current conflicts. *Social Research, 75*(2), 615–655.

Bagozzi, R., & Dabholkar, P. A. (1994). Consumer recycling goals and their effect on decisions to recycle: A means-end chain analysis. *Psychology & Marketing, 11*(4), 313–350.

Bahgat, G. (2004). Oil, terrorism, and weapons of mass destruction: The Libyan diplomatic coup. *Journal of Social, Political & Economic Studies, 29*(4), 373–394.

Bell, J. B. (2002). The organization of Islamic terror: The global Jihad. *Journal of Management Inquiry, 11*(3), 261–268.

Berman, N. (2006). Intervention in a 'divided world': Axes of legitimacy. *European Journal of International Law, 17*(4), 743–769.

Bindra, S. (2001, September 19). India identifies terrorist training camps: Sources told CNN that more than 120 camps are operating in the two countries. *CNN*.

Bjorklund, V. B., Reynoso, J. I., & Hazlett, A. (2005). The anti-terrorist financing guidelines: The impact on international philanthropy. *Pace Law Review, 25*, 233–253.

Borkowski, N. M. (1994). Demarketing of health services. *Journal of Health Care Marketing, 14*(4), 12–22.

Cillufo, F. (2000). *The threat posed from the convergence of organized crime, drug trafficking, and terrorism*. A report delivered before the U.S. House Committee on the Judiciary Subcommittee on Crime, December 13, 200. http://epsilennyt.com/NYTContent/Test/Template33/Images/threadconvergorgancrime.pdf.

Comm, C. L. (1997). Demarketing products which may pose health risks: An example of the tobacco industry. *Health Marketing Quarterly, 15*(1), 95–102.

Crowson, H. M., Debacker, T. K., & Thoma, S. J. (2006). The role of authoritarianism, perceived threat, and need for closure or structure in predicting post-9/11 attitudes and beliefs. *Journal of Social Psychology, 46*(6), 733–751.

Djerejian, E. P. et al. (2003). *Changing minds winning peace*. Report of the Advisory Group on Public Diplomacy for the Arab and Muslim World, October 1, 2003, p. 8.

el-Aswad, el-S. (2012). *Muslim worldviews and everyday lives*. Lanham, MD: Alta Mira Press, Rowman & Littlefield Publisher.

el-Aswad, el-S. (2013). Images of Muslims in Western scholarship and media after 9/11. *Digest of Middle East Studies* (DOMES), *22*(1), 39–56.

Eren, C. S. S. A. (2007). Psychology and the mindset of suicide bombers. In *Suicide as a weapon*. NATO Science for Peace and Security Series, E: Human and Societal Dynamics, Vol. 30, Center of Excellence Defense against Terrorism. Netherlands: IOS Press.

Ersen, U. (2007). Overview of the crisis management related to a terrorist attack. In *Suicide as a weapon*. NATO Science for Peace and Security Series, E: Human and Societal Dynamics, Vol. 30, Center of Excellence Defense against Terrorism. Netherlands: IOS Press.

Esposito, J. L., & Mogahed, D. (2007). *Who speaks for Islam? What a billion Muslims really think*. New York: Gallup Press.

Friedman, T. L. (2007). *The world is flat*. New York: Picador.

Frisble, G. A., Jr. (1980). Demarketing energy: Does psychographics research hold the answer? *Journal of the Academy of Marketing Science, 8*(3), 196–211.

Fullerton, J., & Kendrick, A. (2006). *Advertising's war on terrorism: The story of the U.S. State Department's Shared Values Initiative*. Spokane, WA: Marquette Books.

Gerwehr, S., & Daly, S. (2006). Al-Qaida: Terrorist selection and recruitment. *Homeland Security Handbook*. New York: McGraw-Hill.

Ghaffarzadegan, N. (2008). How a system backfires: Dynamics of redundancy problems in security. *Risk Analysis, 28*(6), 1169–1188.

Glon, J. C. (2005). Good fences make good neighbors: National security and terrorism—Time to fence in our southern border. *Indiana International & Comparative Law Review, 15*, 349–360.

Gundlach, G. T., Bradford, K. D., & Wilkie, W. L. (2010). Counter marketing and demarketing against product diversion: Forensic research in the firearms industry. *Journal of Public Policy and Marketing, 29*(1), 103–122.

Haq, F., Medhekar, A., & Ferdous, T. (2011). Health literacy for muslim consumers: A strategic demarketing approach. *Journal of Global Intelligence and Policy, 4*(4), 54–66. http://search.ebscohost.com/login.aspx?direct=true&AuthType=cookie,ip,url,shib&db=a9h&AN=66211004&site=ehost-live&scope=site. Accessed April 2019.

Hefner, R. W. (2002). Global violence and Indonesian Muslim politics. *American Anthropologist, 104*(3), 754–765.

Hui, J. Y. (2010). The internet in Indonesia: Development and impact of radical websites. *Studies in Conflict & Terrorism, 33*(2), 171–191.

Huntington, S. P. (1993). The clash of civilizations? *Foreign Affairs, 72*(3), 22–49.

Huntington, S. P. (1996). *The clash of civilizations and the remaking of the world order*. New York: Simon & Schuster.

Harvey, M., & Kerin, R. (1977). Perspective on demarketing during the energy crisis. *Journal of the Academy of Marketing Science, 5*(4), 327–338.

Hayes, S. F. (2006, June 16). Saddam's terror training camps. *The Weekly Standard*. http://www.weeklystandard.com/Content/Public/Articles/000/000/006/550kmbzd.asp.

Helms, N. (2009, June 5). Army report: Drug cartels, terrorists infiltrate U.S. *Newsmax.com*. http://www.newsmax.com/Newsfront/mexico-border-fence/2009/06/05/id/330755.

Heuer, R. J. (1999). *The psychology of intelligence analysis*. Central Intelligence Agency: Center for the Study of Intelligence.

Intelligence and Terrorism Information Center. (2009). *The Israeli navy captures a ship carrying a large shipment of weapons*. http://www.terrorism-info.org.il/malam_multimedia/English/eng_n/html/iran_e035.htm.

International Peace Institute. (2016). *The pros & cons of drones in counterterrorism*. Retrieved from https://www.ipinst.org/2016/02/a-terrorist-a-president-and-the-rise-of-the-drone#7 on February 27, 2019.

Kelman, H. C. (1961). Processes of opinion change. *Public Opinion Quarterly, 25,* 57–78.

Karmon, E. (2007). The role of intelligence in combating suicide terrorism. In *Suicide as a weapon*, NATO Science for Peace and Security Series, E: Human and Societal Dynamics, Vol. 30, Center of Excellence Defense against Terrorism. Netherlands: IOS Press.

Klein, P. (2009). International convention for the suppression of financing of terrorism. *United Nations Audiovisual Library of International Law*. http://untreaty.un.org/cod/avl/pdf/ha/icsft/icsft_e.pdf.

Kotler, P., & Levy, S. J. (1971). Demarketing, yes, demarketing. *Harvard Business Review, 79*(6), 74–80.

Laqueur, W. (2000). *The new terrorism: Fanaticism and arms of mass destruction*. Oxford, England: Oxford University Press.

Larobina, M. D., & Pate, R. L. (2009). The impact of terrorism on business. *Journal of Global Business Issues, 3*(1), 147–157.

Lincoln, B. (2006). An early moment in the discourse of terrorism: Reflections on a tale from Marco Polo. *Comparative Studies in Society and History, 48*(2), 242–260.

Lipka, M. (2017, August 9). Muslims and Islam: Key findings in the U.S. and around the world. *Factank: News in the Numbers*. Retrieved from http://www.pewresearch.org/fact-tank/2017/08/09/muslims-and-islam-key-findings-in-the-u-s-and-around-the-world.

Martin, G. (2018). *Understanding terrorism: Challenges, perspectives, and issues* (6th ed.). Los Angeles: Sage Publications.

McCauley, C., & Moskalenko, S. (2011). *Friction: Radicalization happens to them and us*. New York: Oxford University Press.

McCulloch, J., & Pickering, S. (2005). Suppressing the financing of terrorism proliferating state crime, eroding censure and extending neo-colonialism. *The British Journal of Criminology, 45*(4), 470–486.

Munson, H. (2004). Lifting the veil. *Harvard International Review, 25*(4), 20–23.

Naipal, V. S. (1982). *Among the believers, an Islamic journey*. NewYork: First Vintage Books Edition, Random House.

National Commission on Terrorist Attacks Upon the UnitedStates. (2004). *9/11 commission report*. Washington, DC: Government Printing Office.

O'Neill, S. (2009, September 9). Airline bomb plot: Mosque has been recruiting ground for 20 years. *Times Online*. http://www.timesonline.co.uk/tol/news/uk/crime/article6818794.ece.

Peterson, P. G., Bloomgarden, K. F., & Grunwald, H. A. (2003). *Finding America's voice: A strategy for reinvigorating U.S. public diplomacy*. Council on Foreign Relations.

Pieth, M. (2006). Criminalizing the financing of terrorism. *Journal of International Criminal Justice, 4*(5), 1074–1086.

Post, J. M. (2007). *The mind of the terrorist: The psychology of terrorism from the IRA to al-Qaeda*. New York: Palgrave Macmillan.

Rana, M. H., & Malik, M. S. (2016). Human resource management from an Islamic perspective: A contemporary literature review. *International Journal of Islamic and Middle Eastern Finance and Management, 9*(1), 109–124.

Robertson, N., & Cruickshank, P. (2009, November 16). Libyan Group Denounces bin Laden Ideology. *CNN*. http://edition.cnn.com/2009/WORLD/africa/11/16/libya.alqaeda.robertson/index.html.

Sagan, S. D. (2004). The problem of redundancy: Why more nuclear security forces may produce less nuclear security. *Risk Analysis, 24*(4), 935–946.

Samier, E. A. (2017). Islamic public administration tradition: Historical, theoretical and practical dimensions. *Administrative Culture, 18*(1), 53–71.

Shughart, W. F., II. (2006). An analytical history of terrorism: 1945–2000. *Public Choice, 128*(1–2), 7–39.

Skuba, C. J. (2002). Branding America. *Georgetown Journal of International Affairs, 3*(2), 105–114.

Sloan, S. (2002). Meeting the terrorist threat: The localization of counter terrorism intelligence. *Police Practice and Research, 3*(4), 337–345.

Smith, A., & Fitchett, J. A. (2002). The first time I took acid I was in heaven: A consumer research inquiry into youth illicit drug consumption. *Management Decision, 40*(4), 372–383.

Speier, R. H., Chow, B. G., & Starr, S. R. (2001). *Nonproliferation sanctions*. Santa Monica, CA: RAND Distribution Services. http://www.rand.org/pubs/monograph_reports/MR1285/.

Stanton, A. L. (2018). Islamic emoticons and religious authority: Emerging practices, shifting paradigms. *Contemporary Islam, 12*(2), 153–171.

Stern, J. (2010). Mind over martyr: How to deradicalize Islamist extremists. *Foreign Affairs, 89*(1), 95–108.

Tuch, H. N. (1990). *Communicating with the world: U.S. public diplomacy overseas* (p. 3). New York: St. Martin's Press.

U.S. Department of Homeland Security. (2009), *The Internet as a terrorist tool for recruitment and radicalization of youth (White Paper)*. April 24, 2009. http://www.homelandsecurity.org/hsireports/Internet_Radicalization.pdf.

U.S. Department of Homeland Security. (2011). *Ten Years after 9/11: Assessing airport security and preventing a future terrorist attack*. September 16, 2011.

Wall, A. P. (2005). Government demarketing: Different approaches and mixed strategies. *European Journal of Marketing, 39*(5/6), 421–427.

Wall, A. P. (2006). Government 'demarketing' as viewed by its target audience. *Marketing Intelligence & Planning, 25*(2), 123–135.

Wiktorowicz, Q., & Kaltenthaler, K. (2006). The rationality of radical Islam. *Political Science Quarterly, 121*(2), 295–320.

Wright, C. C., & Eagan, J. (2000). De-marketing the car. *Transport Policy, 7*(4), 287–294.

Zangoueinezhad, A., & Moshabaki, A. (2011). Human resource management based on the index of Islamic human development: The Holy Quran's approach. *International Journal of Social Economics, 38*(11–12), 962–972.

Chapter 8
Proposed Response: Counterterrorism Strategies Focusing on the Demand Side of the Terrorism Market

Abstract In this chapter we discuss counterterrorism strategies focusing on the demand side of the terrorism market. We do so by focusing of drivers of market demand: culture, religion, economy, politics, globalization, and media. We propose specific counterterrorism strategies that are directly deduced from our analysis of the drivers of market demand.

Keywords Counterterrorism · Drivers of jihadist terrorism · Culture · Religion · Economy · Politics · Globalization · Media · Communication technologies

8.1 Introduction

> Let us make our future now and let us make our dreams tomorrow's reality.
>
> Malala Yousafzai[1]

This is the final chapter in the book. In this chapter and in the previous chapters we have travelled a path seeking to understand the underlying drivers of Islamist Jihadist terrorism. We have sought to explore this issue, not from a position of total expertise on the topic, but as a group of scholars and citizens of the world who offer some suggestions regarding the framing of the conversation about this plague that has been visited upon all people by those who seek to corrupt the words of God and His Prophets for political gain. This is not to say that there are no foundations for these feelings of anger and retribution brought on by exploitation by any number of political, social, and religious institutions over the past decades, and perhaps centuries. The past is full of stories of exploitation, savagery, and brutality carried out in the name of God. History has taught us, however, that the great religions and nations of the world all hold as their basic tenants, compassion and caring for fellow men and women. Chapter 4 begins with a quote from the Prophet Mohammed that includes as part of the passage "Spread peace among yourselves." The capacity for

---

[1] https://www.brainyquote.com/quotes/malala_yousafzai_569369.

© Springer Nature Switzerland AG 2019   149
M. J. Sirgy et al., *Combatting Jihadist Terrorism through
Nation-Building*, Human Well-Being Research and Policy Making,
https://doi.org/10.1007/978-3-030-17868-0_8

compassion and caring for one's fellow men and women is what the Quality-of-Life directed approach to a demand-side framework embrace. Such an approach is aimed at mitigating the ill-being elements of the underlying causes of Islamist Jihadist terrorism. Obviously, there is no simple answer to the problem, nor is there one that is based on simple short-term fixes focused on treating a variety of visible "news worthy" symptoms. A genuine solution must embrace a wide-spread and multi-faceted treatment program that gets to the root causes of this cancer that is terrorism. It is only through such an approach that Islamist jihadist terrorism can become seen by all Muslims and members of all religions as abhorrent to all professors of faith and true followers of God.

The drive to advance peoples' quality of life is global and adequate social and public policies play a critical role in improving peoples' overall well-being. The objective of this chapter is to show to what extent understanding the drivers of ideologies and activities of jihadism help governments and policy makers generate sociocultural plans and public policies aimed at employing a set of interventions designed to effectively combat the terror of militant jihadists. Policy makers can no longer disregard the threat staged by violent jihadist ideologies and actions, but if they are to be eradicated, they must be identified and understood. Policy strategies and responses to terrorism need to be multi-faceted and efficient. Let's face it, the Islamist jihadist menace is not likely to fade into oblivion soon. See Box 8.1 for recognized patterns and trends.

Box 8.1: The Islamist Jihadist Movement: Patterns, Trends, and Events

- **Islamist jihadist propaganda cannot be prevented**. Islamist militants have discovered the utility of the internet, the global media, and social networking media in spreading their wrapped and extremist beliefs and recruiting new militants.
- **A new generation of Islamist extremists has been primed**. The war in Iraq has created new training and recruitment opportunities for Islamist militants, replacing Afghanistan. Jihadist militants will disperse in various countries including their own home countries. They are likely to pose a major threat to secular governments in the MENA region and the West.
- **Al-Qaeda has become more than an organization; it has evolved to become a symbol and ideology**. Osama bin Laden, founder and leader of Al-Qaeda is viewed as a statesman and an intellectual mouthpiece for Islam. He has become a symbolic mentor for this and future generations of Islamist jihadists. His death has elevated him further—he is viewed as a martyr for Islam.
- **ISIS has become a symbol and inspiration for resurgent violence by Islamist extremists**. Many Muslim scholars view ISIS as an evolution of resurgent Islamist ideology. ISIS's promise is the creation of a new pan-Islamic caliphate. ISIS has managed to recruit thousands of radical Islamists into their ranks. Although the war against ISIS has been successful in the

retaking of territory in Syria and Iraq, ISIS fighters are likely to wage in the same manner of Al-Qaeda militants, namely guerilla warfare.
- **The jihadi movement has become a globalized phenomenon**. Radical Islamists have managed to disseminate information and images about their war to the point of creating solidarity among Islamists. A new cadre of recruits are likely to join the movement, especially young people who live in the West.
- **Christian extremists continue to promote a religious motivation for the war on jihadi terrorism**. Many Christians see the jihadist movement as a war against Judeo-Christianity. This is most evident on Christian websites and comments from Christian leaders and clerics mostly in the United States. They believe that Islamic faith is "evil" and the war on terrorism is a divine plane pitting the true faith (i.e., Judeo-Christianity) against Islam. This increasing rhetoric is likely to increase Islamophobia among Westerners, which may spill over into political overtures that may backfire against the West.

Source: Martin (2018, p. 151).

Terrorism or militant Islamist jihadism is viewed here as a market, with both a supply side and a demand side (Iannaccone, 2006; Krueger, 2007; Stern, 2003). "The requirements for running terrorist organizations are similar to those running a firm" (Stern, 2003, p. 142). The supply side includes economic and opportunity costs. Using market terms, individuals, either in small groups or on their own, supply their services to terrorist organizations for those who demand them (Krueger, 2007).[2] The demand side of the Islamist jihadist terrorism market includes multiple elements such as cultural, ideological, economic, political, and religious drivers, among other factors. The long-term solution to the problem of terrorism and militant religious radicalism lies in changing market conditions, particularly the demand side toward which terrorist organizations aspire to succeed (Iannaccone, 2006). However, the West has largely failed to address the root causes of terrorism. Specifically, the current Western response to Islamist jihadist terrorism has focused on the supply side of the economics equation through dismantling economic resources, finance, funding, and other material capacities of the terrorist groups. But, the demand side of the economics equation has not been given proper attention.

Discussing terrorist activities, Krueger (2003) argues that the main motivation for such activities is deep devotion to a political, social or religious cause. While consideration of economic or opportunity costs is relevant, it is necessary to focus on the demand side not only by degrading terrorist organizations' financial and technical capabilities, but also by designing effective interventions to treat the causes of ill-

---

[2]Another example, terrorist killers are viewed as suppliers of labor, while those who recruit them are the demanders (Iannaccone, 2006).

being that generate terrorism. Additionally, it is important to promote peaceful means of protest, so there is no need for surmounting grievances through violent actions (Krueger, 2007). In brief, policies should target causes rather than consequences. "Groups and societies routinely induce people to kill and die for causes far removed from their personal well-being" (Iannaccone, 2006, p. 10).

This book has attempted to provide a holistic approach about one of the most pressing contemporary public-policy issues and reflects a holistic approach toward the analysis of a wide range of policy frameworks designed to counter terrorism at local, national, regional and international levels. It tackles the underlying ideology shared by the Islamist jihadist groups, as revealed in their activities and propaganda so as to provide effective counter-policies for and from governments and civil society both within and without the Muslim world. Some data tackle the shortcomings or negative elements hindering the realization of wellbeing that scholars and policy makers strive to highlight, decrease and eliminate.

Public policy, intending to affect a vast portion of the public, indicates the process or means through which a government acts to improve people's quality of life or deal with the needs of its citizens via plans and actions as defined by its laws or its constitution (Birkland, 2016; O'Donnell et al., 2014). Social policy, concurrently, refers to the plans or programs designed by the political system and the private sector to solve both the public problems confronting the society and to achieve the objectives pursued by the greater population (el-Aswad, 2019). As shown in subsequent sections, the drivers of well-being and policy issues in Middle Eastern and Muslim countries vary according to the types of government and non-government agencies and actors in each country.

The development of interventions to enhance well-being presupposes that policy makers understand the causes of ill-being that drive or motivate militant jihadists. In other words, if policymakers know what causes ill-being in individuals, families, organizations, or nations, they should be able to use this knowledge to develop effective interventions. Social public policy is expected to improve not only public-sector services but also the relationship between the people and their governments. More efficient policies are needed to improve national security and safety-related wellbeing by increasing budgets for public security provisions to support police operations and state security systems, and to augment the income or salaries of security agents and professionals. Moreover, and additionally, effective policies are required to protect the poor and the vulnerable, including the elderly and the refugees (el-Aswad, 2019) as well as those who may be dissatisfied with the current situation or those suffering from lack of wellbeing. In general, higher public spending on national security and social welfare is associated with higher wellbeing at the national level (Huppert & Cooper, 2014).

8.2 Global Terrorism and Global Response

Most of the studies dealing with terrorism and ill-being do not incorporate adequate measures of terrorism worldwide. According to the Global Terrorism Database (2018), terrorism has escalated over the past decade.[3] For instance, the total number of deaths resulting from terrorism rose from under 10,000 in 2006 to over 32,000 in 2014, reflecting an increase of 287%. Terrorism and internal conflict have been major causes in the global deterioration of peacefulness over the decade. The average level of global peacefulness has dropped for the fourth consecutive year and fell by 0.27% in 2017 (Global Peace Index, 2018).[4] In addition, terrorism has spread around the globe, occurring in both developing and developed or economically prosperous and peaceful countries. The terrorist campaign against the West or the United States and the developed world generally is merely the latest example of a much larger phenomenon. This phenomenon, however, is not a mere political-military threat, rather it is a social-psychological menace caused by grievance and dissatisfaction (Mazarr, 2004).

It is to be noted that 62 % of countries worldwide had terrorism impact scores that deteriorated between 2008 and 2018 (Global Peace Index, 2018). This coincided with the rise of ISIS or the Islamic State of Iraq and the Levant (ISIL) and Boko Haram, intensifying fights and conflicts in the Middle East particularly, and the growing levels of terrorism in the West. Although one hundred countries experienced increased terrorist activity, the Middle East and North Africa (MENA), remained the world's least peaceful region followed by the South Asian region (Global Peace Index, 2018). Table 8.1 shows that five MENA countries are the least peaceful countries in the world. In 2017, terrorist attacks in the Middle East and North African region reached 3,780 (or 35% of the attacks worldwide) out of which 1,321 terrorist attacks were carried out by the ISIL. More than half of all deaths took place in three countries: Iraq (24%), Afghanistan (23%), and Syria (8%) (Study of Terrorism and Responses to Terrorism [START], 2018). "Using Islam as a power ideology is one of the major causes for the fragmentation and division that plague most of the MENA countries. This situation is reflected in the Iran-Iraq War 1980–1988 (Sunni vs. Shi'a) and Iraq's invasion of Kuwait 1990 (Sunni vs. Sunni) as well as in the internal conflict in Libya, Yemen, civil war in Syria, and the boycott of Qatar by Saudi Arabia, the UAE, and Egypt in June 2017 (Salafi and Wahhabi Vs. both Muslim Brotherhood and Shi'a)" (el-Aswad, 2019, p. 39).

The war against terrorism constitutes an imperative factor of the foreign and public policies of many nation-states. On 8 September 2006, the United Nations

---

[3] A recent study shows that "jihadists have recruited more than forty-thousand foreign fighters from 110 countries. Of these, about six-thousand have been U.S., Australian, Canadian, or European Union (EU) nationals travelling to the conflict zones in Iraq and Syria, both before and since the ISIS caliphate declaration of June 2014" (Magen, 2018, p. 111).

[4] Globally, the top five most peaceful countries are Iceland (scoring 1.096), New Zealand (scoring 1.192), Austria (scoring 1.274), Portugal (scoring 1.318), and Denmark (scoring 1.353) (Global Peace Index, 2018).

Table 8.1 Global peace
index of the MENA Countries
(out of 163 Countries), 2018

Regional rank	Global rank	Country	Score
1	42	Kuwait	1.799
2	45	UAE	1.82
3	56	Qatar	1.87
4	71	Morocco	1.979
5	73	Oman	1.984
6	78	Tunisia	1.998
7	98	Jordan	2.104
8	109	Algeria	2.182
9	129	Saudi Arabia	2.417
10	130	Bahrain	2.437
11	131	Iran	2.439
12	141	Palestine	2.621
13	142	Egypt	2.632
14	146	Israel	2.764
15	147	Lebanon	2.778
16	149	Turkey	2.898
17	153	Sudan	3.155
18	157	Libya	3.262
19	158	Yemen	3.305
21	160	Iraq	3.425
22	163	Syria	3.6

Source Data extracted from the Global Peace Index (2018); the
higher the score the lower the peace in that country

General Assembly adopted the Global Counter-Terrorism Strategy operated by the
United Nations Counter-Terrorism Committee. The strategy is an exclusive global
mechanism to augment national, regional and international efforts to individually
and collectively prevent and combat terrorism (United Nations Office of Counter-
Terrorism, 2016). Peace is to be maintained not only within nations, but across nations
by addressing and solving issues related to the social-psychological menace (Mazarr,
2004).

The United Nations' strategy of action includes four major components. First,
addressing the conditions conducive to the spread of terrorism. Second, constructing
measures to prevent and combat terrorism. Third, creating channels to build states'
capacity to prevent and combat terrorism as well as to strengthen the role of the
United Nations system dealing with these issues.

Fourth, establishing criteria to ensure respect for human rights for all and ensuring
the rule of law as the fundamental basis for the fight against terrorism (United Nations
Office of Counter-Terrorism, 2016).

Although each government deals with its own exclusive set of historical, economic, social, political geographic, and cultural conditions; poverty, ignorance, inequality, grievance, flawed ideology and ill-being (as discussed in the previous chapters of this book) are some of the most dangerous drivers or causes of jihadi extremism. The United Nations recommends using its capacities in the domains of conflict prevention, mediation, negotiation, conciliation and peacekeeping to contribute to the successful prevention of terrorism as well as to the strengthening of the global fight against terrorism. Additionally, the United Nations urges the World Health Organization to step up its technical assistance to help nation-states improve their public health systems and to prevent and prepare for possible biological attacks by terrorists. Another operation of global policy can be implemented by reinforcing the cooperation among nation-states in combating crime that might be connected with terrorism, including money laundering, illicit arms trafficking and other potentially lethal and deadly materials (United Nations Office of Counter-Terrorism, 2016).

Several studies have shown that militant Islamist jihadists from different militias and movements such as Al-Qaeda's and ISIL are predominantly recruited from relatively wealthy and well-educated, middle class family backgrounds, most of whom are trained in scientific or technical disciplines (Krueger, 2007; Sageman, 2004, 2008; Scheuer, 2004; Testas, 2004). However, evidence indicates that terrorist organizations thrive where states are economically and politically weak (el-Aswad, 2006, 2016b; Gold, 2004; Helman and Ratner, 2010; Lassalle, 2016; Newman, 2007).

Research dealing with issues of combating global and local terrorism propose that foreign aid is important for inducing local countries with weak governments to fight terrorism within their sphere of influence and sovereignty. Such countries are interested in preemptive joint counter-terrorist operations as well as in the welfare of their population, particularly those living in the war zone. The donor serves as a provider for both development aid and military forces to jointly wage the anti-terrorism war. Within this policy framework, the donor community is allocating aid across countries to provide (among other things) stronger incentives for fighting terrorism to governments facing more militias and militant groups (Azam & Delacroix, 2006; Azam & Thelen, 2008, 2010; Chowdhury & Roy, 2011). However, such military efforts are not completely effective, but rather constitute part of the short-term policy (Habeck, 2006; Sirgy, Estes, & Rahtz, 2017). "Current military efforts to undermine the Islamic State territorial control in such cities as Fallujah, Ramadi, and Mosul have so far done little to ameliorate local grievances, such as anger at the slow pace of reconstruction and the presence of Shi'a militias among the Sunni population. In Libya, improving national and local governance is essential to undermine Salafi-jihadist groups in the long run" (Jones et al., 2018, p. 1). However, establishing an effective governmental system under the current circumstances has proved to be quite challenging.

8.3 Drivers of Terrorism and Proposed Policies of Counterterrorism

By providing policy makers with the necessary information of the drivers and motivations of the jihadists, governments and civil societies can design effective plans and policies to counter terrorism. Terrorism is a socio-political activity driven by group dynamics and motivations in the sense that acts of terrorism are carried out by individuals and small groups, motivated by specific factors and drivers (Shemella, 2002). These factors, discussed in detail in previous chapters, include cultural, religious, ideological, economic, political, and global media drivers. These drivers will be addressed in the following sections within the framework of proposed policies aimed at combating and countering terrorism.

8.3.1 Culture and Counterterrorism Strategies

Culture is a powerful driver for the development and well-being of people.[5] However, under certain circumstances and conditions, any community or society may be inclined to produce a culture of terrorism (el-Aswad, 2016a). Any cultural combat against terrorism is contingent on a clear-cut understanding of the complex relationship between militant jihadists or terrorist groups and their cultural backgrounds. Western-born Muslim jihadists, particularly young people, can be vulnerable to forms of radicalization if they experienced an early identity crisis from attempting to settle the conflicts of feeling irrelevant or disconnected from what the first generation perceived as a Muslim identity while feeling that they are not fully recognized by or integrated with the wider Western society. Moreover, intensified hostility to marginalized Muslim communities in the West can fuel radicalization (el-Aswad, 2008).

The quality-of-life approach proposes that in addition to the history of the Western colonialism of Muslim countries, Western prejudice or discrimination against Muslims and the increased perception of the decadence of Western culture in Muslim societies have a negative impact on aggrieved Muslims and, as a result, trigger violent and terrorist actions carried out by militant jihadists (Sirgy, Estes, & Rahtz, 2017). Moreover, in order to replace contaminated effects of Western culture with a moral one based on Islamic religious values, radical jihadists seek to reinstate the Caliphate or Islamic state in Muslim countries (Sirgy, Joshanloo, & Estes, 2018). As aforementioned, extremist and rigid interpretation of parts or elements of a specific

---

[5]According to Tylor (1871, vol. 1, p. 1), culture "is that complex whole which includes knowledge, beliefs, arts, morals, law, customs, and any other capabilities and habits acquired by man as a member of society." This definition implies that culture, individual and society are inseparable (el-Aswad, 1990). For the United Nations, culture is defined as "the set of distinctive spiritual, material, intellectual and emotional features of a society or a social group" (United Nations Research Institute For Social Development, 2013, p. 12).

culture, religion, or ideology such as the demand to re-establish the Islamic caliphate or participate in the final battle of the apocalypse can be invoked to substantiate or justify radical culture and terrorist acts. "One group's political hero is another group's terrorist and vice versa" (Blain, 2009 p. 13). In short, many jihadist movements target Western countries because the West is viewed as responsible for the plight Muslims encounter.

With respect to counterterrorism, eliminating a terrorist group physically does not dismantle its ideology or change the underlying conditions that permitted the group to commit terrorist actions in the first place. Reconstruction, rehabilitation particularly reconciliation is just as important as any military counterterrorism campaign in building societal resilience against the appeal of terrorism (Wright et al., 2017). Implementations of initiatives and policies aimed at advocating and protecting the dignity of aggrieved Muslims may help reduce Jihadist terrorism.

Internationally, the United Nations' proposed strategies are directed toward denouncing any sort of prejudice or discrimination, promoting a culture of peace, and encouraging mutual respect for cultures, religions, and religious values and beliefs. Such a strategy might increase cultural understanding and rational dialogues between Muslims and non-Muslims, leading to the establishment of effective and peaceful policies (el-Aswad, 2012). Cultural dialogue and engagement within and across local, regional and global communities can lead not only to the annihilation of the adverse influence of militant and extremist groups, but also to the development of proactive security solutions in today's endangered world (United Nations Office of Counter-Terrorism, 2016). Such international policies may yield positive results reducing the western blame and discrimination of Muslims that in turn might reduce the cultural ill-being and negative feelings jihadists have toward the West.

Regionally, the League of Arab States has proposed that partnerships and collaboration in the domains of cultural and educational activities such as conferences and public lectures among other activities that aim to promote values of tolerance and acceptance of the non-violent other are necessary for reducing animosity and improving the quality of life of those in Arab countries (Egypt Today, 2017, League of Arab States, 2018).

Nationally, each MENA government should use well-being research outcomes based on a valid and widely accepted methods to formulate strategic initiatives for the development of cultural policies to sustain and spend on cultural endeavours, including heritage and art, as key drivers toward improving its overall quality of life (el-Aswad, 2019) (Table 8.2).

8.3.2 Religion, Religious Ideology, and Counterterrorism Strategies

According to the quality-of-life approach, religious ill-being drivers are represented in Islamic extreme religiosity and lack of secularism. Extreme religiosity can give rise

Table 8.2 Ill-being drivers of Jihadism and counterterrorism policies

Drivers	Ill-being factors → terrorism	Counterterrorism policies and recommendations
Cultural factors	Perceived decadence of Western culture	Cultural dialogue and mutual respect
	Western prejudice and discrimination against Muslims	Protection and rehabilitation of the dignity of aggrieved Muslims
Religious factors	Increased religiosity and extremism	Advocate religious moderation and expose the danger of extremism
	Lack of secularism in Muslim countries	Promote secularism in Muslim countries via science, technology, arts, and humanities and social sciences
Economic factors	Income inequality-poverty	Reduce inequalities in economic well-being within and across Arab countries
	Unemployment	Create entrepreneurship programs and regional systems of aid and support
		Provide employment opportunities
	Disparities in technological innovation	Promote technological innovation in aggrieved MENA countries
Political	Authoritarian tribal regimes	Decentralize government institutions
	Exclusionary undemocratic systems	Nation-building policies supporting democratic systems and civil liberties
Globalization and Media	Global media bias against Muslims	Establish online media-educational campaigns refuting both islamophobia and terrorism
	Online-media terrorism	

to radicalism and fanaticism as in the case of Islamist Jihadist terrorism. Countries with increased extreme religiosity and decreased secular life are inclined to score lower on the indicators of quality of life than countries with decreased religiosity and increased secularism (Sirgy, Estes, & Rahtz, 2017).

Although Arabism and pan-Arabism, particularly in the 1950s and 1960s, was a popular model for Arabs, it did not prosper because of the interference of global and regional powers and the lack of both democratic systems and effective policies. Since the 1970s, the "ideologization" of Islam or Islamically-oriented ideologies have replaced Arab nationalism and socialism in the Arab world in reaction to the defeat of 1967 war with Israel (el-Aswad, 2019). At the same time, secularism in most Muslim and MENA countries began to significantly decline opening more doors for a swift rise of conservative or hard line Islamist movement, radicalism, and militancy in those countries (el-Aswad, 2016b). In brief, increased religiosity and lack of secularism in Islamic countries play a significant role in incidence of Islamist jihadist terrorism (Sirgy, Estes, & Rahtz, 2017, p. 827).

As opposed to state violence, terrorism is viewed as violence committed by non-state actors (Hoffman, 2017). For young persons, the attraction exerted by Islamist jihadism appears to be motivated by the religiously justified violence it preaches (Mezzetti, 2017; Roy, 2007). Acts of terrorism are carried out by individuals and small groups, driven by specific motivations and factors. These factors include grievance, rage, recognition, revenge, and material gain. However, religion is held responsible as a core element of such factors, even in cases of non-religious uses of terrorism (Juergensmeyer, 2003; Stern, 2003).

Religious ideology, especially of the extremists, can be a very rigid and inflexible system of beliefs that can be leveraged to force people, without offering any sort of compromise, to behave in specific manners. Religious ideology plays a critical role in the terrorist activities of the militant Islamist jihadists. In other words, religious extremists such as the worldwide terrorist activities of al-Qaeda in the name of Islam, have abused the power of the faith by transforming it into a radical ideology to guide destructive behavior (el-Aswad, 2016a).

As stated earlier in this book, religion is hijacked by terrorists and exaggerated or distorted for ideological purposes. In the meantime, while many moderate Muslims, ordinary people as well as leaders, have rejected many aggressive U.S. foreign policies toward certain Muslim countries, they have also rejected bin-Ladin's indiscriminate killing (Beutel & Ahmad, 2011) of others. The majority of al-Qaeda and its ideological associates' victims have been Muslims. For instance, in 2007 the State Department and National Counterterrorism Center found at least 50% of the victims from the attacks of al-Qaeda were Muslims. Such attacks included the targeted damage or destruction of approximately 100 mosques. Other reports have indicated that 85% of al-Qaeda's fatalities occurred in Muslim-majority countries (Beutel & Ahmad, 2011).

It is the fanatic religious mindset to which militant Islamist jihadists have always been tempted and for which the radical dogmatists are ready to offer a framework of blame, hate, violence and totalitarian politics that constitute one of the major causes of the threat people encounter in different places (Mazarr, 2004). Put differently, extreme political ideologies and events are exposed to the pressures of religion and sources of motivation alone cannot drive ordinary citizens to undertake excessive measures against innocent people; they are generally provoked by captivating leaders and encouraged by relatedly motivated partners (Shemella, 2002) as well as situations or conditions of ill-being.

Concerning international policies of counterterrorism, the United Nation's Arab Human Development report (2016) states,

> The overwhelming majority of young people in the Arab region have no desire to become
> radical or to participate in extremist or violent groups or activities. The overwhelming major-
> ity also see religion as distinct from ideology and do not wish for the latter to encroach on the
> former. … However, the minority that accepts violence and is open to participating in violent
> groups that claim to struggle for change continue to be active. (United Nations Development
> Programme, 2016, p. 36)

To counter the minority of young people adopting violence and terror as a way
of struggle for change, the United Nations recommends tackling the conditions conducive to the acceptance of such violent behavior.

Regional cooperation is crucial to ensuring that interventions aimed at refuting
religious extremism are successful. The Organization of Islamic Cooperation (OIC)
establishes policies aimed at promoting moderation or mediation, conflict prevention and resolution, crisis management in member states, and contributions to peace-
building initiatives. In addition, the Organization of Islamic Cooperation and the
United Nations office of counter-terrorism signed a memorandum of understanding
(MoU) on cooperation between the two organizations to counter terrorism. One of
the counterterror policies is to fight extreme forms of religion and to present the true
image of tolerance within Islam (Organization of Islamic Cooperation, 2018a). The
Organization of Islamic Cooperation "firmly rejects the identification of terrorism
with any nationality or religion and has always highlighted the necessity of addressing the conditions that foster terrorism by promoting human rights, tolerance and
multiculturalism and tackling negative socio- economic factors" (Organization of
Islamic Cooperation, 2017).

Moderate Muslim leaders need to lead their congregations into exploring the true
teachings of Islam in relation to such extreme behavior and, in turn, must become
active spokespersons leading the way for peace and harmony between Muslims and
others (Sirgy, Estes, & Rahtz, 2017). MENA governments should develop educational
policies to enhance citizens' appreciation of the value of secularism. This can be done
through education at both primary and secondary levels. In order to help reduce
Islamist jihadist terrorism government officials and policy makers should develop
programs that promote secularism in Muslim countries, particularly those that suffer
from terrorist attacks. It is to be noted that Alex Schmid (2017) states that moderate
Muslims are committed to secularism and moderation stands for tolerance, freedom,
compassion, justice and peace. Moderate Muslims must develop alternative methods
opposing the literalist interpretation of Islam. The more people become well-versed in
science/technology and arts/humanities, the more likely they become less religiously-
obsessed (Sirgy, Estes, & Rahtz, 2017).

At both national and local levels, counterterrorism and attempts to confront and
undermine militant extremism are bound to fail if they do not work to nullify the
Islamist jihadist religious ideology.[6] Put differently, the end of Islamist jihadist religious ideology might be expected to indicate the end of jihadist terrorism (Gregg,
2010). But, to end militant Islamist jihadism, a new strategy or policy is needed to
counter the ideology of Islamic extremism. More efforts are required to uncover the

---

[6]See Chap. 5 in this book.

weaknesses and contradictions inherent in the religious ideologies of militant jihadist groups as well as in their improper use of Islamic principles and values. For example, one of the weakest points in the jihadist ideology is the drive to kill Muslim people who belong to different sects or adopt different ideas. Therefore, efforts to counter a corrupted jihadist religious ideology can succeed from within the ideological communities. Groups driven by ideology normally have strong leadership (el-Aswad, 2013). Often being perceived as a symbol of their organization, jihadist terrorist leaders take important positions in their groups and beyond. It is therefore important that counter-terrorism strategies target the leadership of terrorist organizations (van Leeuwen and Weggemans, 2018).

Government officials and policy makers should develop policies aimed at changing the framework of Muslim extremists' religiosity and militancy. Militant jihadist leaders need to be challenged by moderate Muslim leaders who are expected to be able to display the discrepancies and gaps between extremists' religious ideologies and actions as well as the contradictions between religious propaganda of different jihadi groups (el-Aswad, 2016a). Moderate Muslim leaders should work to challenge the influence of the religious interpretations of militant jihadists by promoting the moderate interpretations of Islamic texts. For example, the relationship between Islam and political order "had been weakened by modern leaders of Islamic countries, such as those in … Egypt" (Juergensmeyer, 2003, p. 65).

Countering Islamist jihadist ideological preaching (da'wa) is considered an important long-term strategy because extremists rely on and manipulate it for recruiting members and gaining sympathy and support from young people (Habeck, 2006). It is to be noted that open religious markets incite religious moderation by encouraging and facilitating the entry and involvement of numerous competing religious groups. Militant theologies or ideologies, for instance, "are most effectively neutralized by competing theologies, which are in turn most effectively produced by competing religious groups" (Iannaccone, 2006, p. 17) (Table 8.2).

8.3.3 Economic Ill-Being and Counterterrorism Strategies

The economic drivers of terrorism imply economic ill-being factors that include income disparities, poverty, and unemployment, on the one hand, and low levels of technological innovation, on the other (Sirgy, Estes, & Rahtz, 2017). Globally, the economic impact of violence increased by two per cent during 2017 due to a rise in the socio-economic impact of conflict and increases in internal security spending (Global Peace Index, 2018). To the contrary, the Global Peace Index (GPI) report found that peacefulness has a considerable impact on macroeconomic performance. In the last 70 years, per capita growth has been three times higher in highly peaceful countries when compared to countries with low levels of peace. The difference is even stronger when looking at changes in peacefulness, with the GPI report finding that per capita GDP growth has been seven times higher over the last decade in countries that improved in peacefulness versus those that declined and deteriorated (Global

Peace Index, 2018). Unstable socioeconomic and psychological factors are intimately interrelated. But, the former becomes precarious when joined to the latter (Mazarr, 2004). Although poverty alone does not create or explain terrorism (Krueger, 2003; Krueger and Maleckova, 2003; Gold, 2004), deprived and unhappy people, living in a disrupted environment, can be vulnerable and dangerous to the rest of society (Shemella, 2002).

With regard to counterterrorism policies, the United Nations has proposed that cultural activities, public goods, and sectors such as trade, education, sustainable cultural tourism, and cultural infrastructure can serve as strategic mechanisms for peace and non-violence advocacy as well as for revenue generation, particularly in developing countries, given their rich cultural heritage and substantial labor force (UNESCO, 2012; World Bank, 2001, 2015). In addition, Western democracies, which are the main targets of terrorist attacks, should invest more funds in foreign aid with a special emphasis on supporting technological training and education (Azam & Thelen, 2008).

Success in the war against terror requires a multi-pronged approach involving not only counter-terror operations, but also developmental aid (Chowdhury & Roy, 2011). At the regional level, the Arab League should embrace long-term policies focusing on improving peaceful human capital as well as on eliminating inequalities in economic well-being within and across Arab countries. Moreover, the Arab League should establish regional systems of aid and support that would meet and sponsor the needs of victims of terrorism and their families and help the rehabilitation of their lives. Nationally or locally, if Islamist terrorism is viewed as a market enticing potential employees to pursue careers in terrorism (Krueger, 2007), leading to negative consequences, it is wise that governments or public and private sectors create other more appealing and productive options of employment. Additionally in order to alleviate economic deprivation, policy makers and governments must provide well designed policy issues to ensure employment opportunities for the unemployed, particularly among the young who represent about 30% of the total population of MENA region (el-Aswad, 2019; Keulertz et al., 2016). Such economic policies may reduce the grievance of the deprived and decrease the option of using terrorist actions. Policy makers also must address the sources of resentment to be found within militant Muslims. Appropriate compensation and training can reduce corruption among government employees and security forces and help convey a sense of fairness in dealings with the public.

Governments should promote identity-seeking through commerce, support investment, scholarship plans to international programs, and other means of developing and encouraging entrepreneurship as conventionally understood in the West (Mazarr, 2004). Public policies and programs should focus on promoting technological innovation in aggrieved MENA countries so as to promote secularism, improve communication and education, and enhance personal quality of life in an effort to reduce the incidence of Jihadist terrorism (Sirgy, Estes, & Rahtz, 2017).

8.3.4   Political Ill-Being and Counterterrorism Strategies

Social policy is a profoundly political process of sociocultural production shaped by social actors in different locations who exert remarkable amounts of influence. These actors differ in their authority to define what is problematic in well-being, shape the explanations and mechanisms of how problems of terrorism should be resolved, and determine how the image of future change efforts should be directed (el-Aswad, 2019). This study proposes a call for democratization of the Middle East governments as well as a request for endorsing and encouraging specific reform advocates and Muslim leaders of movements trying to bring greater accountability to their countries (el-Aswad, 2019). Policy makers and political authorities should support and promote tolerant models of government in Muslim majority countries that work against extremism.

Political ill-being drivers pertaining to terrorism refer to factors of authoritarian, tribal, and exclusionary regimes. Long -lasting authoritarian, tribal, repressive and exclusionary regimes in most Muslim and Middle East countries have a critical impact on the negative sentiments of aggrieved Muslims, leading to the grave incidence of Islamist Jihadist terrorism. (Sirgy, Estes, & Rahtz, 2017). Terrorist attacks increase in repressive regimes when the political situation is not moving in a direction the militant jihadists prefer, regardless of economic incentives (Krueger, 2003). Countries with authoritarian regimes score lower on indicators of quality of life than countries with democratic regimes. It is interesting to note that in several cases the West has supported authoritative, repressive and corrupt regimes in the MENA region (el-Aswad, 2008). Insofar as jihadist political ideology blames authoritarian and corrupt rulers for the plight of Muslim countries, the policy of counter Islamist jihadist ideology should initiate a plan informing or advising Western governments not to support such corrupt and repressive regimes (Koppman, 2015).

Terrorism is a political form of violence and counterterrorism is its political response. "The terrorist is fundamentally a *violent intellectual*, prepared to use and, indeed, committed to use force in the attainment of his or her goals" (Hoffman, 2017 p. 20 emphasis in the original). Scholarly accounts suggest that terrorists, motivated by geopolitical grievances, are concerned with influencing political outcomes. In essence, the contention is that those who embrace strong political views are assertive enough to impose an extremist viewpoint by violent means (Krueger, 2007). Policy makers must offer comprehensive and cognizant views or options to neutralize the jihadist appeal for the most politically vulnerable targets including organizations, institutions and persons. As noted earlier, it is interesting to point out that the United Nations and the League of Arab States have agreed to develop joint activities, such as seminars, workshops, trainings, projects and other initiatives, to build the capacity of members of the Arab League in the fields of counterterrorism and prevention of violent extremism (United Nations, 2018).

Internationally, the United Nations' counterterrorism plan addresses underlying conditions such as the political, social and economic marginalization that leads to terrorist actions worldwide (United Nations Office of Counter-Terrorism, 2016). The international community should encourage authoritarian regimes to establish democratic and civil principles through education and diplomatic means asserting human rights (Sirgy, Estes, & Rahtz, 2017). International data show a positive relationship between democratic institutions and life satisfaction, including the extent to which individuals participate in referenda. In advanced industrial democracies life satisfaction is related to the extent of state intervention to protect citizens against pure market forces, controlling for economic, social, cultural, and individual-level factors. This relationship is held across diverse income levels and political ideologies (Huppert & Cooper, 2014).

Nationally and locally, governments in the MENA region should assert the pre-eminence of human rights and reaffirm the importance of international law (Sirgy, Estes, & Rahtz, 2017). National problems cannot be solved by violence or terrorism, but rather by scientific and rational means in a democratic environment. However, governments alone cannot defeat terrorist groups. The society itself must take the initiative to counter ideologies and actions of militant jihadism and terrorism. Civil society and non-government organizations (NGO) play a critical part in confronting and weakening the militant jihadism. It is also government's responsibility to establish a healthy environment for the civil society to heal itself. A good example of the role of civil society confronting terrorism is represented in the tribesmen activities and actions in Al Anbar region, in Iraq, where tribal forces, directed by the government, managed to remove the ISIS terrorists from that region (Shemella, 2002).

Nation-states with low levels of civil liberties are more likely to be the countries adopting fanatics and perpetrators of terrorist attacks (Krueger, 2007). When freedom of expression and other civil liberties are protected, violent ways of reaction will cease. Support for, and the defense of civil society should be part of the preventive policy in the war against terrorism (Krueger, 2003). Local leaders should help those who have returned from fighting with militant groups in order to discredit the extreme jihadi ideology. To ensure the existence of a healthy and active civil society, government authorities must promote civil liberties and encourage local leaders to provide appropriate advice and guide to the young people alerting them about the danger of all forms of extremism (Shemella, 2002) (see Table 8.2).

Some of the most critical policies that need to be implemented are to decentralize government institutions, to increase life satisfaction, and help people become happy through employment and identity-seeking entrepreneurship. Moreover, government and NOG institutions should adopt policies that encourage and support Muslim reformers to oppose violence in any form, domestic and/or international. More efforts are needed to support public and political policies that provide initiatives to solve geopolitical conflicts and political instability across the MENA region especially for those experiencing instability and strife (el-Aswad, 2019). To put it another way, it is important to reach a fair resolution of the conflict zones in the Middle East, particularly the Israel-Palestine conflict that triggers much of the terrorist actions not only in the Middle East region, but also in Western countries (el-Aswad, 2019; Habeck, 2006).

All in all, comprehensive social-public policy plans are needed to activate civil society by launching national and regional programs that motivate people to actively engage and participate in public life and civic initiatives. It is important for policy makers to support dynamic and strong private, informal sectors as well as to encourage stakeholders to participate in policy processes that can reduce conflicts and create environment of peace for people, particularly the youth (male and female) in the MENA region. One of the significant and positive roles of culture is represented in its contribution to knowledge, education, and politics. Cultural heritage, cultural art, and cultural creative industries can serve as strategic mechanisms for peace and non-violence advocacy (UNESCO, 2012).

8.3.5 Globalization, Media and Communication Technologies

Globalization and media ill-being factors affecting terrorism are represented in the global or Western media bias toward Muslim countries contributing to the rise of the negative sentiment of aggrieved Muslims (Sirgy, Estes, & Rahtz, 2017). The problem is that Western media have portrayed the majority of Muslims in terms of global terrorism, Islamic jihadism, Islamism, fascism, and authoritarianism creating what is known as Islamophobia or an irrational fear of Muslims. "These global depictions of Muslims … have not only aggravated sociopolitical problems in the Arab/Muslim world such as poverty, unemployment, homelessness, violence, and the 'brain drain' caused by migration but have also led to serious questions concerning indigenous cultures, identities of Muslim diaspora" (el-Aswad, 2013, p. 41). The Muslim public in the MENA region and other Muslim countries have become exposed to Western decadence through the global media. For example, Hillary Clinton, in a documented YouTube video (2016), admitted twice in public that the U.S. government fights the jihadists it created 20 years ago. The U.S. government created Al-Qaeda and recruited the *mujahedin* in 1980s to fight the Soviet Union in Afghanistan, and then, after defeating the Soviet Union, left these trained fighters, who were fanatical and well-armed, in Afghanistan, Pakistan and Arab countries.

Islamist jihadists rely heavily on communication technologies and networks for spreading their propaganda and ideology. Social media allows groups in isolated areas to know about Islamist jihadist's activities as well as to financially support them (Nakhla, 2016).[7] Terrorists' social media and violent acts appear to extremists as the most efficient and cost-effective means of getting a message through. As noted in Chap. 6, Al-Qaeda has put together a truly impressive media infrastructure to support its members and promote itself to potential recruits. Ciovacco (2009). The global village created by the modern media and the Internet means that never before have terrorist acts gained such public prominence (el-Aswad, 2014a, 2014b). Moreover, large numbers of Islamist militant jihadist groups have been recruited through existing social networks including online connections (Sageman, 2004). In the West, Jihadism is more likely to be attractive to young people because the

---

[7]Nakhla (2016) provided diverse case studies of militant jihadists who were sanctioned by UN and US for using social media to publicize messages from and to extremist and terrorist groups.

language its propaganda skillfully makes use of is the one of digital natives which are more familiar and more included in the specific communication (Mezzetti, 2017). Consequently, in the process of countering Islamicist jihadist ideologies and actions, media and propaganda are critical in securing good outcomes (Payne, 2009). With regard to counterterrorism policies, the United Nations supports the Human Rights Council and contributes to its work on the promotion and protection of human rights for all in the fight against terrorism. Further, the United Nations recommends using the Internet as a tool for countering the spread of terrorism, while recognizing that States may require assistance in this regard (United Nations Office of Counter-Terrorism, 2016).

Policies and programs that publicize political, cultural, scientific, and technological achievements, particularly in global media, are valuable means for reducing the threat of Islamist jihadist terrorism (Sirgy, Estes, & Rahtz, 2017). Use of communication technologies such as the Internet, mobile phones, Facebook, Twitter, and YouTube have had significant impact on socioeconomic activities and civil society in MENA countries (el-Aswad, 2014b, 2014c). There has been significant progress in this domain where Internet penetration in the MENA region reached 64.5% of the population in 2017 compared to the worldwide average of 54.5% (Internet World Stats, 2018). Three MENA countries are included in the top 20 nations of Internet users worldwide as of the year 2017: Iran (ranked 17), Turkey (ranked 18), and Egypt (ranked 20) (Internet World Stats, 2018). Specific institutions of Islamic care and counselling (public and private) have created web sites and online services broadly reaching clients and receivers in the MENA region. These web sites allow people comprising a large number of online consumers in the MENA countries to partake freely in discussing certain aspects of health and wellbeing (el-Aswad, 2017a, 2017b).

In its fight against the vicious campaign against Islam, the Organization of Islamic Cooperation initiates media plans projecting the true image of tolerance and noble values of Islam (Organization of Islamic Cooperation 2018b). Muslim intellectuals and activists are involved in transnational missionary work. They strive to construct positive images of Muslims at both national and global levels through public lectures, sermons, conferences, workshops, and media programs (el-Aswad, 2003, 2013). Much of the substance of Muslim worldviews is discussed, reproduced in new forms, and represented in various online Muslim virtual communities (el-Aswad, 2013). Such global activities and activism are planned to undermine and weaken both the islamophobia, manufactured by global media, and propaganda of the Islamist jihadi extremists and terrorists. It is important to start a mutually respectful dialogue with Islamic leaders preaching personal empowerment and nonviolence (Mazarr, 2004).

At the national or local level, governments should apply mechanisms of interventions that confront terrorist ideology by focusing on education and training. It is necessary to improve the quality of education at all levels by increasing funding, updating curricula, boosting administrative systems, recruiting and training highly qualified instructors, and building reliable educational facilities (el-Aswad, 2019). In addition, there is need for advanced technological skills, increased collaboration among stakeholders, enhanced support for weaker and disabled students, and provision of reliable transport and school food options (el-Aswad, 2019) (see Table 8.2). Furthermore, educators can be urged to establish relevant and directed educational campaigns to encourage their audience to refrain from participating in terrorist activities as well as to provide practical advice to prevent people, particularly the young generation, from being attracted to terrorism.

8.4   Conclusion

Within the quality-of-life framework, this research has tackled cultural, religious, economic, political and global media factors underlying drivers of jihadist terrorism in order to provide long-term counterterrorism policies and recommendations aimed at not merely reducing or annihilating terrorism regionally and globally, but also emasculating the acceptability of violence as a tool for achieving political goals. Policy makers, nationally, regionally and internationally, will not be able to create long-term policies to fight terrorism without defining and confronting the broader drivers and causes of militant jihadism. Policymakers and government officials need to better understand the explicit political and other drivers and factors that have allowed militant Salafi-jihadist groups like the Islamic State (or ISIS) and al-Qaeda among other non-state groups to establish regional and global terror bases.

   In addition to the author's recommendations, the study has addressed counterterrorism policies and interventions provided by international, regional and national institutions such as the United Nations, the Arab League, and the Organization of Islamic Cooperation. For example, the inquiry has pointed out that the United Nations has moved way from short-term policies concerning the war on terror, in term of military and other coercive alternatives of the response, to focus on such issues as growing ethnic discrimination against Muslims, slow economic development (in the MENA region), rising unemployment (particularly among educated youth), limited political freedom, the mounting void between the people and the state, political exclusion, the lack of democracy and the abuse of human rights that constitute some of the most critical enticing extreme radicalization and terrorism.

   It is important "for policy-makers and the public to keep an eye on proportions, neither under—nor over—estimating problems: while there are some 1.6 billion Muslims in the world, there are probably not more than 100,000 terrorists in the world who explicitly profess to be engaged in this form of political violence in the name of Islam. Based on this, the ratio of Muslim terrorists—non-violent Muslims would be 1:16,000" (Schmid, 2017, p. 4).

   Regionally, despite the serious efforts for improving people's quality of life, Middle East and North African countries have favoured short-term political stability, security and regime maintenance at the expense of long-term and more progressive political reforms and the development of the institutions necessary to promote the levels of democratic governance, respect for human rights and the rule of law needed to prevent conditions leading to terrorism.

Government authorities should focus not only on terrorists and suspected bombers but on the religious-political ideology and infrastructure required to launch and sustain terrorist and suicide campaigns (Hoffman, 2017). Both local or regional and global counterterror agencies should propose policies and initiatives to attack and criticize the core points at which jihadists' ideology distorts Islamic doctrinal principles and values so as to effectively undermine the entire jihadi extreme religious-political ideology. This particular strategy, however, necessitates the assistance of moderate Muslim leaders.

Militant Islamist jihadism is a complex phenomenon, and a broad array of policies are needed to fight it. Such policies include cultural, ideological, political, economic, and social issues as well as diplomacy and security, among other initiatives. Policy makers should look at the majority, who are politically moderate and advocate mediation. Mediation means the ability of a concept, object, or action to occupy a middle point between two distant or opposite poles. "This notion of mediation is associated with "moderation" (*waṣaṭiyyah*), a fundamental principle of Islam indicating a balance or midway between two extreme ways or positions. The Qur'an proclaims that the Muslim community is a middle [balanced] community. Moderation proves to be practical in social interaction" (el-Aswad, 2012, p. 147).[8] Moderate Muslim leaders must be encouraged to use media networks such as television, radio, newspapers, and magazines as well as cyber communication including online forums, videos, Internet and talk-show to challenge the misleading propaganda of fanatic and militant jihadists.

This book addresses terrorism or militant jihadism as a market, with a supply side and a demand side. The study has focused on the demand side of the Jihadist terrorism's market that includes manifold constituents such as cultural, ideological, economic, political, and religious drivers, among other factors. Within this framework, radical jihadists are less likely to thrive, nor will they adopt violence when there is resilient competition in their markets, particularly in the demand side that requires long-term policies oriented toward preventive or preemptive policies that embrace strategies aimed at competing with the ideologies of extremist jihadism.

In addition to the discussion of strategies concerning cultural, ideological, economic, and political divers, the study addresses other important policy issues related to media, communication technologies, religion and religious leaders, education, and civil society or civil liberty (Table 8.2). The following are the main recommendations addressed in this chapter:

- Support the United Nations' efforts and capacities in the domains of conflict prevention, mediation, conciliation and peacekeeping that contribute to the successful prevention of terrorism.
- Reinforce the cooperation among nation-states in the global fight against terrorism.
- Advocate cultural dialogue, mutual respect and positive engagement within and across local, regional and global communities necessary for the development of proactive security solutions in dealing with the danger of terrorism.

---

[8]"Thus, we have appointed you a middle community [*ummah waṣaṭ*]" (Qur'an 2:143).

- Provide initiatives and policies aimed at protecting the dignity of aggrieved Muslims that, in turn, help reduce Jihadist terrorism.
- More efforts are demanded to expose the contradictions inherent in the religious ideologies of militant jihadist groups that improperly use Islamic principles and values for achieving political goals.
- It is important to reach a fair resolution of the conflict zones in the Middle East, particularly the Israel-Palestine conflict that triggers much of the terrorist actions regionally and globally.
- The MENA region governments and the Arab League should improve the economic quality of life through developing a wide variety of projects that can employ a significant portion of the population, particularly young people. Such a progressive economic policy will encourage young people to stay in the MENA region rather than risk the precarious migration to Western or European countries.
- Policy makers and political authorities should initiate nation-building policies that support democratic life and civil liberty in Middle East and Muslim majority countries as there is a positive relationship between democratic institutions and life satisfaction.
- Endorse cultural and educational activities such as conferences, public lectures, and workshops among other activities that aim to promote values of tolerance and non-violence as effective means for reducing animosity and aggression between people.
- Initiate policies adopting and advancing secularism through science, technology, arts, humanities and social sciences in MENA countries.
- Advance proper and effective use of different forms and networks of global media to confront the ideologies and actions of militant jihadists.

Finally, this book has proposed that a better understanding of the drivers and determinants of ill-being and the dangerous ideology of militant jihadists will provide scholars, policy makers and government officials with relevant considerations and recommendations concerning policy issues necessary for combating terrorism. In ending our endeavour, we hope that decision makers and any other interested parties who have explored our framework and discussion have broadened their understanding of the Islamist jihadist drivers and possible ways to mitigate this scourge upon our world. We pray for all who follow the great religions of the world to remember that all the Prophets have stressed there is a path to peace and understanding that begins with love and caring for each other. Hate ultimately destroys us all.[9]

---

[9]"Hate is too great a burden to bear. It injures the hater more than it injures the hated." https://www.brainyquote.com/quotes/coretta_scott_king_141009.

References

Azam, J.-P., & Delacroix, A. (2006). Aid and the delegated fight against terrorism. *Review of Development Economics, 10*(2), 330–344.

Azam, J. P., & Thelen, V. (2008). The roles of foreign aid and education in the war on terror. *Public Choice, 135,* 375–397. https://doi.org/10.1007/s11127-007-9268-4.

Azam, J. P., & Thelen, V. (2010). Foreign aid vs. military intervention in the war on terror. *Journal of Conflict Resolution, 54,* 237–261.

Beutel, A. J., & Ahmad, I. (2011). Examining Bin Ladin's statements: A quantitative content analysis from 1996 to 2011. *Minaret of Freedom Institute.* Retrieved from https://www.linkedin.com/pulse/examining-bin-ladins-statements-quantitative-content-pj-wilcox.

Birkland, T. A. (2016). *An introduction to the policy process: Theories, concepts, and models of public policy making.* New York: Routledge.

Blain, M. (2009). *The sociology of terrorism: Studies in power, subjection, and victimage ritual.* Boca Raton, Fla.: Universal Publishers.

Barrett, R. (2017). Beyond the caliphate: Foreign fighters and the threat of returnees. *Soufan Center.* Retrieved from http://thesoufancenter.org/wp-content/uploads/2017/11/Beyond-the-Caliphate-Foreign-Fighters-and-the-Threat-of-Returnees-TSC-Report-October-2017-v3.pdf.

Chowdhury, P. R., & Roy, J. (2011). Aid in times of terror. Discussion paper. *Indian Statistical Institute.* Retrieved from file:///Users/elaswad/Downloads/Aid_in_Times_of_Terror.pdf.

Christmann, K. (2012). *Preventing religious radicalization and violent extremism. A systematic review of the research evidence.* Youth Justice Board. Retrieved from https://www.gov.uk/government/publications/preventing-religious-radicalisation-and-violent-extremism.

Ciovacco, C. J. (2009). The contours of Al Qaeda's media strategy. *Studies in Conflict & Terrorism, 32*(10), 853–875.

el-Aswad, el-S. (1990). *Ath-thaqāfah wa att-fkīr: ru'iyah anthropolojiyyah* (Culture and thought: An anthropological view). *The National Review of Social Sciences, Cairo, 27*(3):71–104.

el-Aswad, el-S. (2003). Sanctified cosmology: Maintaining Muslim identity with globalism. *Journal of Social Affairs* (20), 65–94.

el-Aswad, el-S. (2006). The permeability of the Middle East: The predicament of regional and global forces. *Digest of Middle East Studies (DOMES), 15*(1), 113–120.

el-Aswad, el-S. (2008). Al-istishrāq al-jadīd: Jadaliyyat al-thunā'iyya al-thaqāfiyya bayn al-gharb/al-sharq wa al-gharb/al-Islam (New Orientalism: A dialect of cultural dualism between West/East and West/Islam). *Thaqāfāt* (University of Bahrain Press)*, 21,* 204–233.

el-Aswad, el-S. (2012). *Muslim worldviews and everyday lives.* Lanham, MD: Alta Mira Press, Rowman & Littlefield Publisher.

el-Aswad, el-S. (2013). Images of Muslims in Western scholarship and media after 9/11. *Digest of Middle East Studies (DOMES), 22*(1), 39–56. https://doi.org/10.1111/dome.12010.

el-Aswad, el-S. (2014a). E-folklore and cyber-communication among Emirati youth. *International Journal of Intangible Heritage, 9,* 49–62.

el-Aswad, el-S. (2014b). Communication. In K. Harvey (Ed.), *Encyclopedia of social media and politics* (vol. 1, pp. 304–308). Thousand Oaks, CA: Sage.

el-Aswad, el-S. (2014c). Social Worlds. In K. Harvey (Ed.), *Encyclopedia of social media and politics* (vol. 1, pp. 1190–1192). Thousand Oaks, CA: Sage.

el-Aswad, el-S. (2016a). Political challenges confronting the Islamic world. In H. Tiliouine & R. J. Estes (Eds.), *The state of social progress of Islamic societies: Social, economic, political, and ideological challenges* (pp. 361–377). Cham, Switzerland: Springer International Publishing. doi:https://doi.org/10.1007/978-3-319-24774-8_16.

el-Aswad, el-S. (2016b). State, nation and Islamism in contemporary Egypt: An anthropological perspective. *Urban Anthropology, 45*(1–2), 63–92.

el-Aswad, el-S. (2017a). Islamic care and counseling. In D. A. Leeming, (Ed.), *Encyclopedia of psychology and religion* (pp. 1–14). Berlin/Heidelberg: Springer-Verlag.

el-Aswad, el-S. (2017b). Empathy and emerging worldviews. In D. A. Leeming (Ed.), *Encyclopedia of psychology and religion*. Germany: Springer-Verlag GmbH. doi:https://doi.org/10.1007/978-3-642-27771-9.

el-Aswad, el-S. (2019). *The quality of life and policy issues among the Middle East and North African Countries*. New York: Springer Nature Switzerland AG.

Egypt Today. (2017). Arab League adopts Egyptian resolution to develop Arab counterterrorism system. Retrieved from http://www.egypttoday.com/Article/1/35686/Arab-League-adopts-Egyptian-resolution-to-develop-Arab-counterterrorism-system.

Global Peace Index. (2018). *Measuring peace in a complex world*. Retrieved from http://visionofhumanity.org/app/uploads/2018/06/Global-Peace-Index-2018-2.pdf.

Global Terrorism Database. (2018). *Codebook: Inclusion criteria and variables*. Retrieved from https://www.start.umd.edu/gtd/downloads/Codebook.pdf.

Gold, D. (2004). The economics of terrorism. *The New School Graduate Program in International Affairs*. Retrieved from https://www.files.ethz.ch/isn/10698/doc_10729_290_en.pdf.

Gregg, H. S. (2010). Fighting the Jihad of the pen: countering revolutionary Islam's ideology. *Terrorism and Political Violence, 22*(2), 292–314. https://doi.org/10.1080/09546551003597584. Retrieved from https://www.tandfonline.com/doi/abs/10.1080/09546551003597584.

Habeck, M. (2006). *Knowing the enemy: Jihadist ideology and the war on terror*. New Haven: Yale University Press.

Helman, G. B., & Ratner, S. R. (2010). Saving failed states. *Foreign Policy, 89*(1992–1993), 3–20. Retrieved from https://foreignpolicy.com/2010/06/15/saving-failed-states/.

Hoffman, B. (2017). *Inside terrorism*. New York: Columbia University Press.

Huppert, F. A., & Cooper, C. L. (2014). *Interventions and policies to enhance wellbeing: A complete reference guide* (Vol. VI). Chichester, West Sussex: Wiley.

Iannaccone, L. (2006). The market for martyrs. *Interdisciplinary Journal of Research on Religion, 2*(4), 1–14.

Internet World Stats. (2018). *Top 20 countries with the highest number of Internet users 2017*. Retrieved from https://www.internetworldstats.com/top20.htm.

Jones, S. G., et al. (2018). The evolution of the Salafi-Jihadist threat: Current and future challenges from the Islamic State, al-Qaeda, and other groups. *Center for Strategic & and International Studies* (CIS). Retrieved from https://www.csis.org/analysis/evolution-salafi-jihadist-threat.

Juergensmeyer, M. (2003). *Terror in the mind of God: The global rise of religious violence*. Oakland, California: University of California Press.

Kean, G. T. H., et al. (2018). *Digital counterterrorism: Fighting jihadists online*. Retrieved from https://bipartisanpolicy.org/wp-content/uploads/2018/03/BPC-National-Security-Digital-Counterterrorism.pdf.

Keulertz, M., et al. (2016). Material factors for the MENA Region: Data sources, trends and drivers. *Middle East and North Africa Regional Architecture*. Retrieved from https://www.cidob.org/content/download/65695/2014964/version/12/file/MENARA%20Concep%20paper%203_16.pdf.

Koppman, S. (2015, May 6). Endless U.S. support for dictators' powers Islamic state. *Huff-Post*. Retrieved from https://www.huffingtonpost.com/steve-koppman/endless-us-support-for-di_b_6821136.html.

Krueger, A. B. (2003, May 29). Economic scene; cash rewards and poverty alone do not explain terrorism. *New York Times*. Retrieved from https://www.nytimes.com/2003/05/29/business/economic-scene-cash-rewards-and-poverty-alone-do-not-explain-terrorism.html. (Business section).

Krueger, A. B. (2007). *What makes a terrorist: Economics and the roots of terrorism*. Princeton: Princeton University Press.

Krueger, A. B., & Maleckova, J. (2003). Education, poverty and terrorism: Is there a causal connection? *Journal of Economic Perspectives, 17*(4), 119–144. Retrieved from http://www.sas.rochester.edu/psc/clarke/214/Krueger03.pdf

Lassalle, K. E. Ö. (2016). State failure and the political violence phenomenon: A comparative Analysis of Iraq and Syria cases. *European Journal of Interdisciplinary Studies, 2*(2), 168–175. Retrieved from http://journals.euser.org/files/articles/ejis_jan_apr_16/Eylem.pdf

League of Arab States. (2018). *Arab league counterterrorism committee*. Retrieved from https://pilac.law.harvard.edu/multi-regional-efforts//counterterrorism-committee-of-the-league-of-arab-states-arab-league

Macdonald, S. (2018, June 26). How tech companies are successfully disrupting terrorist social media activity. *The Conversation*. Retrieved from http://theconversation.com/how-tech-companies-are-successfully-disrupting-terrorist-social-media-activity-98594.

Magen, A. (2018). Fighting terrorism: The democracy advantage. *Journal of Democracy, 29*(1), 111–125.

Martin, G. (2018). *Understanding terrorism: Challenges, perspectives, and issues* (6th ed.). Los Angeles: Sage Publications.

Mazarr, M. (2004, June/July). The psychological sources of Islamic terrorism: Alienation and identity in the Arab world. *Policy Review, 125.*

Mezzetti, G. (2017). Contemporary jihadism: A generational phenomenon. *Fondazione ISMU.* Retrieved from http://www.ismu.org/wp-content/uploads/2017/07/Mezzetti_Paper_Jihadism_July2017.pdf.

Nakhla, M. (2016). Terrorist financing & social media. *The Camstoll Group, United Nations.* Retrieved from https://www.un.org/sc/ctc/wp-content/uploads/2016/12/TCG_Social-Media-TF_11DEC161.pdf.

Newman, E. (2007). Weak states, state failure, and terrorism. *Terrorism and Political Violence, 19*(4), 463–488.

O'Donnell, G., et al. (2014). *Wellbeing and policy. [Technical report]*. London: Legatum Institute. Retrieved from https://li.com/docs/default-source/commission-on-wellbeing-and-policy/commission-on-wellbeing-and-policy-report—march-2014-pdf.pdf.

Organization of Islamic Cooperation. (2017). *Counter terrorism strategies should be compliant with international human rights laws*. Retrieved from https://www.oic-oci.org/topic/?t_id=13519&ref=5895&lan=en.

Organization of Islamic Cooperation. (2018a). *The OIC signs MoU with the United Nations office of counter-terrorism (UNOCT)*. Retrieved from https://www.oic-oci.org/topic/?t_id=20034&ref=11485&lan=en.

Organization of Islamic Cooperation. (2018b). *Convention of the organization of the Islamic conference on combating international terrorism*. Retrieved from http://webcache.googleusercontent.com/search?q=cache:ics01uXoHGsJ:www.oic-cdpu.org/en/getdoc/%3FdID%3D13+&cd=12&hl=en&ct=clnk&gl=us&client=safari.

Payne, K. (2009). Winning the battle of ideas: propaganda, ideology, and terror. *Studies in Conflict & Terrorism, 32*(2), 109–128. https://doi.org/10.1080/10576100802627738. Retrieved from https://www.tandfonline.com/doi/abs/10.1080/10576100802627738.

Rougier, B. (2007). *Everyday Jihad: The rise of militant Islam among Palestinians in Lebanon* (P. Ghazaleh, Trans.). Cambridge, MA: Harvard University Press.

Roy, O. (2007). The Islamic terrorist radicalization in Europe. In S. Amghhar, A. Boubekeur, & M. Emerson (Eds.), *European Islam: Challenges for society and public policy* (pp. 52–60). Brussels: Center for European Policy Study.

Sageman, M. (2004). *Understanding terror networks*. Philadelphia: University of Pennsylvania Press.

Sageman, M. (2008). Jihad and 21st century terrorism. *Presentation at the New America Foundation.* Retrieved from http://www.youtube.com/watch?v=mWcH5sDHzPQ.

Scheuer, M. (2004). *Imperial hubris: Why the West is losing the war on terror*. Washington, D.C.: Brassey's Inc.

Shemella, P. (2002). Reducing ideological support for terrorism. *Policy Review, 114.* Retrieved from https://www.hsdl.org/?view&did=36080.

Schmid, A. P. (2017). Moderate Muslims and Islamist terrorism: Between denial and resistance. *International Research Center for Counter-Terrorism*. Retrieved from https://icct.nl/wp-content/uploads/2017/08/ICCT-Schmid-Moderate-Muslims-and-Islamist-Terrorism-Aug-2017-1.pdf.

Sirgy, M. J., Estes, R. J., & Rahtz, D. (2017). Combatting jihadist terrorism: A quality-of-life perspective. *Applied Research in Quality of Life, 29*(3), 461–469.

Sirgy, M. J., Joshanloo, M., & Estes, R. J. (2018). The global challenge of jihadist terrorism: A quality-of-life model. *Social Indicators Research*. Retrieved from https://doi.org/10.1007/s11205-017-1831-x.

Stern, J. (2003). *Terror in the name of God: Why religious militants kill*. New York: Harper Collins.

Study of Terrorism and Responses to Terrorism. (2018). *Global terrorism in 2017*. Retrieved from https://www.start.umd.edu/pubs/START_GTD_Overview2017_July2018.pdf.

Testas, A. (2004). Determinants of terrorism in the Muslim world: An empirical cross-sectional analysis. *Terrorism and Political Violence, 16*(2), 253–273.

Tylor, E. B. (1871). *Primitive culture: Researches in the development of mythology, philosophy, religion, language, art and custom* (2 vols.). London: J. Murray.

UNESCO. (2012). *Culture: A driver and an enabler of sustainable development: Thematic Think Piece. UN system task team on the post-2015 UN development agenda*. Retrieved from http://www.un.org/millenniumgoals/pdf/Think%20Pieces/2_culture.pdf.

United Nations. (2018). UN and League of Arab States ink pact to partner on counter-terrorism. *United Nations peacekeeping*. Retrieved from https://peacekeeping.un.org/en/un-and-league-of-arab-states-ink-pact-to-partner-counter-terrorism.

United Nations Development Programme. (2016). *Arab human development report 2016: Youth and the prospects for human development in a changing reality*. Retrieved from http://www.arab-hdr.org/reports/2016/english/AHDR2016En.pdf.

United Nations Office of Counter-Terrorism. (2016). *UN global counter-terrorism strategy*. Retrieved from https://www.un.org/counterterrorism/ctitf/en/un-global-counter-terrorism-strategy.

United Nations Research Institute for Social Development. (2013). *Social drivers of sustainable development*. Retrieved from http://www.unrisd.org/social-drivers-note.

van Leeuwen, L., & Weggemans, D. (2018). Characteristics of Jihadist terrorist leaders: A quantitative approach. *Perspectives on Terrorism, 12*(4), 55–67. Retrieved from https://www.universiteitleiden.nl/binaries/content/assets/customsites/perspectives-on-terrorism/2018/issue-4/04—leeuwen-en-weggemans.pdf.

Wright et al. (2017). *The jihadi threat: ISIS, al-Qaeda and beyond*. Retrieved from https://www.usip.org/sites/default/files/The-Jihadi-Threat-ISIS-Al-Qaeda-and-Beyond.pdf.

World Bank. (2001). *Cultural heritage and development: A framework for action in the Middle East and North Africa*. Washington, DC: Orientations in Development series. Retrieved from https://openknowledge.worldbank.org/handle/10986/13908.

World Bank. (2015). *Our new strategy*. Retrieved from http://www.worldbank.org/en/region/mena/brief/our-new-strategy.

YouTube. (2016). Hillary Clinton admits America created, funded and armed Al Qaeda/ISIS terrorists. Retrieved from https://www.youtube.com/watch?v=FsIp1TDwFLs.

Zalman, A. (2018). Top major causes and motivations of terrorism. *ThoughtCo*. Retrieved from https://www.thoughtco.com/the-causes-of-terrorism-3209053.

The manufacturer's authorised representative in the EU is Springer
Nature Customer Service Centre GmbH, Europaplatz 3, 69115 Heidelberg,
Germany. If you have any concerns regarding our products, please
contact ProductSafety@springernature.com

Printed and bound by CPI Group (UK) Ltd, Croydon, CR0 4YY
29/04/2026
02099455-0002